Fridge, Forks, and Fresh Starts: Building a Healthy Kitchen

Apostle Paula Ferguson

Published by FOSA Publishing LLC, 2025.

FRIDGE, FORKS, AND FRESH STARTS: BUILDING A HEALTHY KITCHEN

First edition. October 7, 2025.

ISBN: 979-8992834451

Written by Apostle Paula Ferguson.

Table of Contents

Acknowledgment of the Journey Ahead

Many people desire to live healthier lives, but too often, they struggle to maintain those habits long-term. The reality is that **achieving a healthy lifestyle is about more than just making good food choices—it's about preparation, access to the right tools, and the environment where those choices are made.** Without a properly equipped kitchen, even the best intentions can fall short.

This book was written to **address the hidden challenges** that prevent people from achieving sustainable health—challenges like limited budgets, shared spaces, and the lack of proper equipment for preparing nutritious meals. **If you don't have the tools to prepare healthy food, how can you maintain a healthy life?** For example, juicing without a juicer becomes frustrating and costly, leading to burnout. By breaking down these barriers, this book empowers readers to transform their kitchens into spaces that support wellness from the inside out.

As someone committed to **helping the body of Christ thrive in all areas—spirit, soul, and body**—I believe that health is a key part of fulfilling God's purpose for our lives. **How we care for our bodies reflects how we honor the gifts God has given us.** This book provides both practical advice and actionable steps to help readers create a kitchen environment that makes healthy living possible, affordable, and sustainable.

Ultimately, this book is about **equipping readers for success**. It's not just about what you eat—it's about setting up your life to support your goals. **Fridge, Forks, and Fresh Starts** was written to help you lay the foundation for a healthy lifestyle that lasts, so you can live fully, serve boldly, and thrive in every area of life.

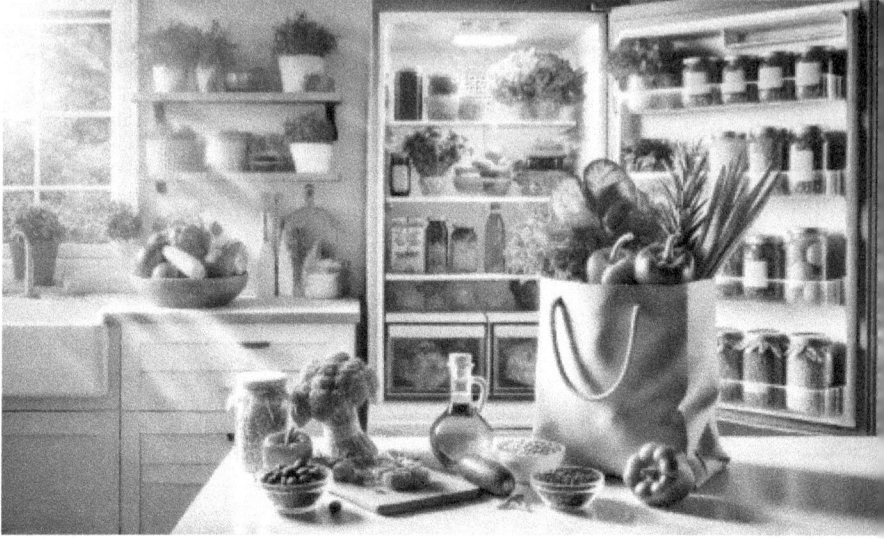

Chapter 1: What is a Healthy Kitchen?

Introduction: It's More Than Just Cutting Sugar

Many people begin their health journey with ambitious declarations: "I'm giving up sugar!" or "No more bread!" But often, these efforts falter because the environment—the kitchen—is still packed with temptations. A healthy kitchen isn't just about eliminating "bad" foods; it's about creating a space that supports your goals and makes healthy choices easy and enjoyable. Whether you live alone or with others, the heart of your lifestyle change begins here, with your kitchen.

This chapter will dive deep into what makes a kitchen "healthy," exploring not just what you stock in it, but how you set it up, manage your environment, and plan for success.

What Does a Healthy Kitchen Look Like?

A healthy kitchen is an environment that promotes mindful, nutritious eating. It helps remove barriers to good choices and reduces reliance on willpower. Here's a breakdown of the key elements:

1. **Accessibility:** Healthy foods are visible and easy to reach. Processed snacks are either absent or hidden.

1. **Balanced Stocking:** You have a variety of whole foods available—fresh fruits, vegetables, lean proteins, whole grains, and healthy fats.

1. **Supportive Tools:** The appliances, utensils, and tools you use promote healthy meal prep and discourage reliance on takeout or packaged foods.

1. **Mindful Design:** The layout encourages cooking and experimenting with healthy recipes, turning meal prep into an enjoyable experience.

Creating this space is the first step toward sustainable change. It's not just about clearing shelves but about filling them with purpose.

Setting Realistic Goals: A Gradual Transition

One of the biggest mistakes people make when building a healthy kitchen is trying to change everything overnight. Sustainable success comes from gradual adjustments, which allow time to adapt both mentally and financially.

Steps Toward Transitioning:

- **Step 1:** Identify the top 3 things in your kitchen that don't align with your health goals (e.g., sugary cereals, sodas, or instant ramen).

- **Step 2:** Create a list of affordable alternatives (e.g., oats for sugary cereals, sparkling water for soda).

- **Step 3:** Plan a weekly or biweekly "swap-out" routine—every payday or grocery run, replace a few items with healthier versions.

Practical Tips to Remove Temptation (Without Feeling Deprived)

Out of sight, out of mind. Research shows that we're more likely to eat what's easily accessible. For example, having a bowl of fruit on the counter makes you more inclined to grab an apple instead of chips. Here are tips to manage temptations effectively:

- **Clear your counters:** Remove processed foods and snacks from visible areas.

- **Create a "treat zone":** If you can't eliminate all indulgent items (especially if you live with others), designate a high shelf or hard-to-reach cabinet for them.

- **Organize your fridge and pantry:** Keep healthy foods front and center—pre-cut veggies, washed fruits, yogurt, and hummus for quick access.

Creating Your Healthy Kitchen Environment

The environment you create determines how easy or difficult it will be to stick to your goals. These adjustments help promote healthy choices every day.

Pantry Essentials for a Healthy Kitchen:

- **Whole Grains:** Quinoa, oats, brown rice, whole wheat pasta

- **Canned Goods:** Beans, lentils, chickpeas, tomatoes (low sodium)

- **Healthy Snacks:** Nuts, seeds, dried fruits (without added sugar)

- **Cooking Oils:** Olive oil, avocado oil, coconut oil

- **Spices & Herbs:** Turmeric, cinnamon, oregano, basil, garlic powder

Fridge and Freezer Essentials:

- **Fresh Vegetables:** Kale, spinach, broccoli, carrots

- **Lean Proteins:** Chicken, turkey, tofu, eggs

- **Dairy Alternatives:** Almond milk, oat milk, yogurt (low sugar)

- **Frozen Fruits and Vegetables:** Great for smoothies and soups when fresh produce isn't available

These staples form the backbone of a balanced kitchen, allowing you to prepare nutritious meals without stress.

How to Build a Healthy Kitchen on a Budget

Building a healthy kitchen doesn't mean breaking the bank. Start small and focus on foods that offer maximum nutrition for the lowest cost.

- **Batch Cooking and Freezing:** Cook large portions of stews, soups, or casseroles and freeze for later.

- **Use Seasonal Produce:** Fruits and vegetables in season are cheaper and often more flavorful.

- **Look for Store Brands:** Many store brands offer high-quality whole foods at a fraction of the cost.

- **Buy in Bulk:** Purchase grains, nuts, and beans from bulk sections to save money.

The Psychology of a Healthy Kitchen: Environment Shapes Behavior

Studies show that the way your kitchen is organized influences your eating habits. If junk food is easily accessible, even the most disciplined person will struggle to resist it. A healthy kitchen isn't just about the food; it's also about how your environment helps reinforce positive behavior.

Here's how environment plays a role:

- **Visual Cues:** When healthy options are front and center, they're more likely to be eaten.

- **Ease of Use:** If nutritious ingredients are pre-prepped and ready to eat, you're more likely to reach for them.

- **Portion Control:** Use smaller plates and bowls to prevent overeating.

Common Pitfalls and How to Avoid Them

It's easy to make mistakes when creating a healthy kitchen, especially if you try to change everything at once. Here are some common challenges and strategies to overcome them:

1. **The Overhaul Mentality:** Don't feel the need to discard everything

overnight. Gradual changes are more sustainable.

1. **All-or-Nothing Thinking:** Allow for some indulgences to avoid feeling deprived.

1. **Overbuying Healthy Foods:** Start with a realistic shopping list to avoid food waste.

1. **Ignoring the Importance of Preparation:** Plan meals ahead and pre-prep ingredients to make healthy eating easier.

Resources to Help You Get Started

Here are some helpful tools and resources to support your healthy kitchen journey:

- **Meal Planning Apps:** PlateJoy, Paprika, or Yummly

- **Budget Shopping Guides:** Use the *USDA Seasonal Produce Guide* to find affordable fruits and veggies

- **Cookbooks for Healthy Eating:**

- *How Not to Die Cookbook* by Michael Greger

- *The Healthy Meal Prep Cookbook* by Toby Amidor

- **Online Communities:** Join Facebook groups or subreddits like r/EatCheapAndHealthy for inspiration

- **YouTube Channels:** Follow chefs and nutritionists for meal ideas (e.g., Downshiftology, Clean & Delicious)

Conclusion: The First Step Toward Change Starts in the Kitchen

Creating a healthy kitchen is the foundation of a sustainable lifestyle. It's not about drastic changes, but about setting yourself up for success by making small, meaningful shifts. Your kitchen should be a place that inspires you to eat well and take care of yourself, not one filled with guilt or temptations.

Whether you're starting on a budget or going all in, the key to success lies in intentional planning and gradual adjustments. Begin by identifying areas for improvement, swap out unhealthy items for nutritious alternatives, and organize your kitchen to encourage healthy habits. As you move forward, each small change will bring you closer to the life you envision—a life of wellness, energy, and joy.

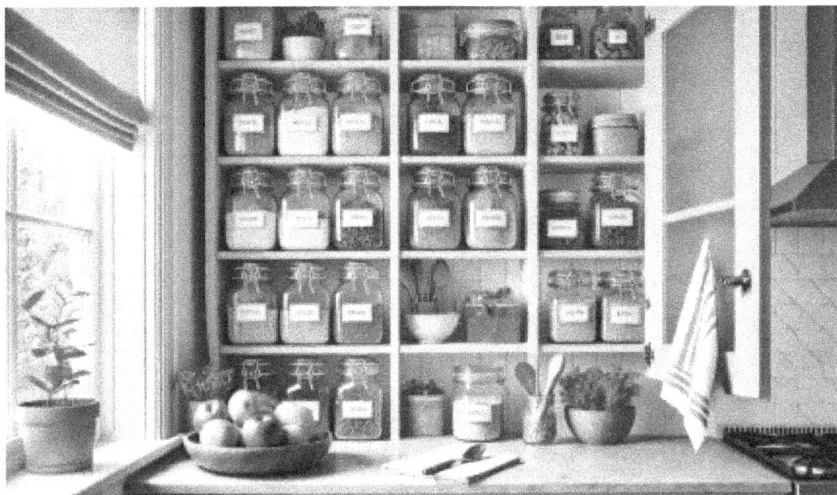

Chapter 2: How to Transition to a Healthy Kitchen on a Budget

Introduction: The Myth That Healthy Eating is Too Expensive

A common misconception about healthy living is that it's only for people with unlimited resources. But with planning, strategy, and intentional choices, anyone can transition to a healthy kitchen on a budget. This chapter focuses on practical, actionable advice to help you replace unhealthy foods and habits while staying mindful of your financial limits. You don't need to overhaul your entire kitchen overnight; slow and steady wins the race.

Step 1: Assess What You Already Have

Before heading to the store, start by assessing your current pantry, fridge, and freezer. It's easy to overlook what you already have and buy more than you need, which wastes both food and money. Here are the steps to take:

- **Inventory Check:** Make a list of all the staples in your kitchen—grains, canned goods, frozen items, and spices.

- **Identify Hidden Gems:** Often, healthy items like beans, oats, or frozen vegetables are tucked behind less healthy ones. Bring these to the forefront.

- **Use What You Have:** Commit to creating a few meals from existing pantry items to prevent waste and free up space for healthier alternatives.

Step 2: Plan Affordable Swaps and Gradual Changes

Replacing unhealthy foods all at once can be overwhelming, both mentally and financially. A more sustainable strategy is to make small swaps over time.

Examples of Healthy, Affordable Swaps:

- **White Bread → Whole Wheat Bread:** Look for store brands or buy in bulk.

- **Sugary Cereal → Oats or Granola:** Oats are versatile, filling, and much cheaper.

- **Soda → Sparkling Water or Infused Water:** Use lemons, berries, or mint to flavor water.

- **Snack Bars → Homemade Energy Bites:** Use oats, peanut butter, and honey to make easy no-bake treats.

- **Chips → Popcorn or Nuts:** Air-popped popcorn is an affordable snack with fewer additives.

Gradual changes make it easier to adjust your taste buds and habits without feeling deprived.

Step 3: Master the Art of Meal Planning and Budgeting

Meal planning is essential to avoid overspending or falling back into old eating habits. Here's a simple approach to planning meals on a budget:

1. **Start With a Weekly Plan:** Map out 4-5 meals that you can rotate throughout the week.

1. **Use Ingredients in Multiple Ways:** For example, roasted vegetables can be used in salads, wraps, or grain bowls.

1. **Batch Cooking:** Prepare large portions of meals and freeze them in individual servings. This reduces waste and saves time.

1. **Repurpose Leftovers:** Turn dinner leftovers into next-day lunches.

Tools for Meal Planning on a Budget:

- **Meal Prep Apps:** Try apps like Paprika, Mealime, or Prepear for planning meals and generating shopping lists.

- **Budget Calculators:** Use tools like Mint or Goodbudget to track your grocery expenses.

Step 4: Affordable Pantry Staples to Build a Healthy Kitchen

Filling your pantry with inexpensive, healthy ingredients helps ensure you always have the basics to make nutritious meals.

Affordable Pantry Staples:

- **Grains:** Brown rice, quinoa, oats, whole wheat pasta

- **Legumes:** Canned or dry beans, lentils, chickpeas

- **Nuts & Seeds:** Peanuts, sunflower seeds, chia seeds

- **Canned Goods:** Diced tomatoes, coconut milk, broth (low sodium)

- **Seasonings:** Salt, pepper, garlic powder, Italian seasoning

Bonus Tip: If your budget allows, buy staples in bulk to save money over time. Many grocery stores and co-ops have bulk sections where you can stock up on essentials.

Step 5: Make the Most of Seasonal Produce

Buying fresh fruits and vegetables in season is an excellent way to save money. Produce that is in season is often more affordable, tastier, and more nutritious.

Examples of Seasonal Savings:

- **Fall:** Apples, squash, sweet potatoes

- **Winter:** Citrus fruits, Brussels sprouts, kale

- **Spring:** Asparagus, strawberries, peas

- **Summer:** Tomatoes, zucchini, berries

Check out the **USDA Seasonal Produce Guide** to help you plan grocery trips based on what's in season.

Step 6: Smart Shopping Strategies for Tight Budgets

Grocery shopping on a budget requires strategy. Here are some tips to get the most out of every trip:

- **Make a List and Stick to It:** Impulse buying is one of the biggest ways to blow your budget.

- **Shop the Perimeter:** The healthiest foods (produce, dairy, and meats) are usually located around the perimeter of the store.

- **Use Store Apps:** Many grocery chains have apps with digital coupons and special discounts.

- **Buy Frozen Produce:** Frozen fruits and vegetables are often cheaper than fresh and have a longer shelf life.

- **Shop Late in the Day:** Many stores discount perishable items toward the end of the day.

Step 7: Incorporate Inexpensive Homemade Meals

Cooking at home is usually cheaper than dining out. Here are a few meal ideas that are both affordable and nutritious:

- **Vegetable Stir-Fry:** Use frozen vegetables and serve over brown rice or quinoa.

- **Lentil Soup:** Lentils are inexpensive and loaded with protein. Add carrots, onions, and spices for flavor.

- **Overnight Oats:** Mix oats with almond milk and top with fruit and nuts.

- **Egg Scramble:** Eggs are an affordable source of protein. Add vegetables and whole grain toast on the side.

How to Navigate Eating Healthy When Living With Others

If you share your home with family, roommates, or a partner, sticking to your healthy kitchen goals can be challenging. Here are some strategies to navigate shared spaces:

1. **Create Your Own Section:** Dedicate a shelf or a drawer for your healthy foods.

1. **Communicate Your Goals:** Let others know about your intentions so they can support you.

1. **Find Common Ground:** Identify healthy foods that everyone enjoys to encourage shared meals.

1. **Compromise on Treats:** Agree to limit the number of unhealthy snacks kept in common areas.

Making the Most of Limited Kitchen Equipment

If your budget doesn't allow for fancy gadgets, don't worry! You can prepare healthy meals with just a few essential tools:

- **Basic Tools:** A good knife, cutting board, and mixing bowls are all you need to start.

- **Slow Cooker or Instant Pot:** These appliances are perfect for batch cooking on a budget.

- **Blender:** Use for smoothies, soups, and sauces (look for refurbished models if you're on a budget).

- **Reusable Containers:** Great for storing leftovers and meal preps.

Free and Low-Cost Resources for Healthy Eating

Building a healthy kitchen on a budget is easier with the right resources. Here are some free or affordable options:

- **Local Food Banks:** Many food banks provide fresh produce and other healthy options.

- **Farmer's Markets:** Some markets offer discounts or accept SNAP benefits.

- **Community Cooking Classes:** Check if your local library or community center offers free classes.

- **Online Recipes:** Websites like Budget Bytes and Minimalist Baker focus on healthy, affordable meals.

- **Public Health Programs:** Some health departments offer free nutrition counseling.

The Power of Planning and Persistence

Building a healthy kitchen on a budget requires patience and persistence. The key is to start small, plan ahead, and make adjustments as you go. You don't need a perfect kitchen to begin eating healthier—you just need a plan and a willingness to take the first step.

Conclusion: It's Possible to Create a Healthy Kitchen, Even on a Budget

A healthy kitchen isn't reserved for the wealthy—it's achievable for anyone with the right mindset and strategies. By planning ahead, making gradual changes, and prioritizing affordable whole foods, you can build a kitchen that supports your health goals without breaking the bank.

The transition may take time, but every small change brings you closer to a sustainable, healthy lifestyle. In the next chapter, we'll explore how to navigate shared kitchens and maintain your healthy eating habits when living with family or roommates.

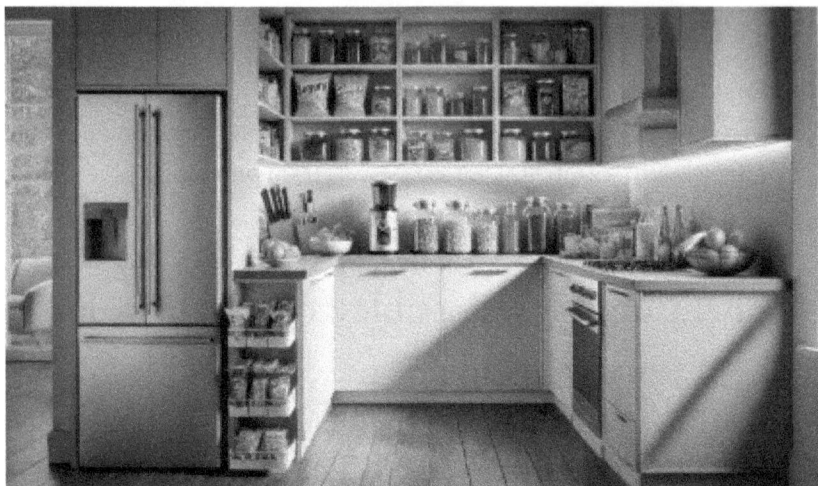

Chapter 3: Healthy Kitchens When You Don't Live Alone

Introduction: Navigating Shared Spaces Without Losing Sight of Your Goals

Living alone makes it easier to maintain control over what food is in your kitchen, but many people share their home with family members, roommates, or a partner. Each person has different eating habits and preferences, which can make it difficult to stick to your health goals. In this chapter, we'll explore practical strategies for navigating shared spaces and fostering a positive food environment—even when the people you live with aren't on the same health journey.

Step 1: Establish Clear Communication About Food Boundaries

Open communication is crucial when transitioning to a healthier lifestyle, especially in a shared kitchen. Whether you're living with family, a partner, or roommates, the way you talk about your health goals can impact their response.

Tips for Clear Communication:

- **Share Your Why:** Explain your motivation to adopt healthier habits (e.g., better energy, health concerns, or fitness goals).

- **Avoid Judgment:** Focus on your choices without criticizing the eating habits of others.

- **Ask for Support, Not Permission:** Let them know how they can help you succeed, such as limiting treats in shared spaces.

- **Negotiate:** Compromise on what can be shared or stored in common areas to avoid conflict.

Step 2: Design Your Own "Healthy Zone" in the Kitchen

When you share a kitchen, one effective strategy is to carve out a space specifically for your healthy items. This helps keep your nutritious options organized and makes them easy to access.

Ideas for Creating Your Healthy Zone:

- **Fridge Space:** Use a designated shelf for your prepped veggies, yogurt, and meal prep containers.

- **Pantry Space:** Dedicate a bin or a section for your healthy snacks, grains, and canned goods.

- **Freezer Space:** Store smoothie packs, frozen veggies, and batch-cooked meals in labeled containers.

- **Visual Cues:** Keep your healthy foods within easy reach, and use opaque containers to store tempting treats.

Step 3: Manage Different Eating Styles Without Conflict

It's common to live with people who may not share your commitment to healthy eating. Instead of creating tension, look for ways to blend your eating styles and introduce healthy habits in subtle ways.

Practical Tips for Coexisting Peacefully:

- **Offer Healthy Alternatives:** If your family loves chips, try introducing air-popped popcorn as an alternative.

- **Cook Together Occasionally:** Find recipes everyone enjoys to encourage healthy meals.

- **Respect Differences:** Allow occasional indulgences, but keep them out of your healthy zone.

- **Lead by Example:** When others see your positive changes (e.g., better energy or weight loss), they may be inspired to join you.

Step 4: Healthy Eating with Kids in the House

Introducing healthy eating to children can be challenging, but building healthy habits from an early age sets them up for long-term success.

Strategies for Encouraging Healthy Eating in Kids:

- **Involve Them in Meal Prep:** Let children help with age-appropriate tasks in the kitchen.

- **Make Healthy Snacks Fun:** Offer fruit kabobs, yogurt parfaits, or "ants on a log" (celery, peanut butter, and raisins).

- **Don't Ban Treats Completely:** Allow occasional treats to prevent feelings of deprivation.

- **Set a Good Example:** Kids are more likely to eat what they see you eating.

Step 5: How to Handle Temptations in Shared Spaces

Living with people who keep unhealthy snacks around can make it harder to stick to your goals. Here are strategies to help you manage these temptations:

- **Create Physical Barriers:** Store tempting treats in opaque containers or on high shelves.

- **Out of Sight, Out of Mind:** Ask others to keep their indulgences in personal cabinets or drawers.

- **Have Healthy Replacements Ready:** When cravings strike, reach for a healthier option (e.g., fruit, nuts, or yogurt).

- **Practice Mindful Eating:** If you indulge, enjoy the treat mindfully to avoid overeating.

Step 6: Meal Planning for Mixed Households

It can be challenging to plan meals for people with different preferences, but there are ways to ensure that everyone is satisfied without compromising your goals.

Ideas for Healthy Meals That Please Everyone:

- **Build-Your-Own Meals:** Taco nights, grain bowls, or salad bars allow everyone to customize their plates.

- **Modify Recipes:** Prepare the same meal but make slight adjustments (e.g., make whole-grain pasta for you and regular pasta for others).

- **Plan Family Favorites with a Twist:** Make healthier versions of comfort foods (e.g., baked chicken tenders or veggie-loaded spaghetti).

Step 7: Setting Boundaries Without Creating Resentment

Setting boundaries is essential, especially if your household isn't entirely on board with your health goals. The key is to strike a balance between honoring your personal choices and respecting others' preferences.

Examples of Healthy Boundaries:

- **Designate One Treat Night per Week:** This creates structure without complete restriction.

- **Request Respect for Your Space:** Ask others not to leave their treats in your healthy zone.

- **Set Limits on Eating Out:** If family members love fast food, set a limit on how often you participate.

Step 8: Practical Tools for Organizing Shared Kitchens

Shared kitchens can quickly become cluttered and disorganized, making it harder to stick to your healthy eating plan. Use these tools to keep things organized:

Helpful Organization Tools:

- **Clear Bins and Labels:** Keep your healthy foods neatly organized in clear bins.

- **Mason Jars:** Store grains, nuts, and seeds in glass jars for easy access.

- **Meal Prep Containers:** Use stackable containers to store leftovers and batch-cooked meals.

- **Lazy Susans:** Use turntables to maximize space in crowded pantries or fridges.

Resources for Managing Healthy Eating in Shared Spaces

Here are some helpful resources to support your healthy kitchen journey:

- **Books on Family Nutrition:**

- *Raising Healthy Eaters* by Jill Castle

- *The Family Cooks* by Laurie David

- **Meal Planning Apps:** Cozi Family Organizer, Mealime

- **Support Groups:** Join online communities focused on healthy family eating (e.g., Healthy Family Project).

- **Storage Solutions:** Check out The Container Store or IKEA for affordable kitchen organization products.

How to Stay Consistent When Life Gets Busy

Living with others often means dealing with unexpected events—school functions, work stress, or last-minute takeout orders. Here are some strategies to stay consistent:

- **Batch Cook on Weekends:** Prepare large meals on the weekend to have healthy options throughout the week.

- **Create a Snack Station:** Stock a bin with healthy snacks for quick grabs.

- **Practice Flexibility:** Allow for occasional indulgences without guilt.

- **Stay Accountable:** Use a food journal or app to track your progress.

Conclusion: Navigating Shared Spaces for Long-Term Success

Creating a healthy kitchen while living with others requires planning, compromise, and patience. It's important to set realistic boundaries, organize your space, and communicate your goals effectively. By leading by example and introducing small, positive changes, you can maintain your healthy habits without creating tension. Over time, those around you may even be inspired to join your journey.

In the next chapter, we'll explore the tools, appliances, and utensils that can make your kitchen even more conducive to healthy living. From blenders to air fryers, we'll show you what's worth investing in and what's not.

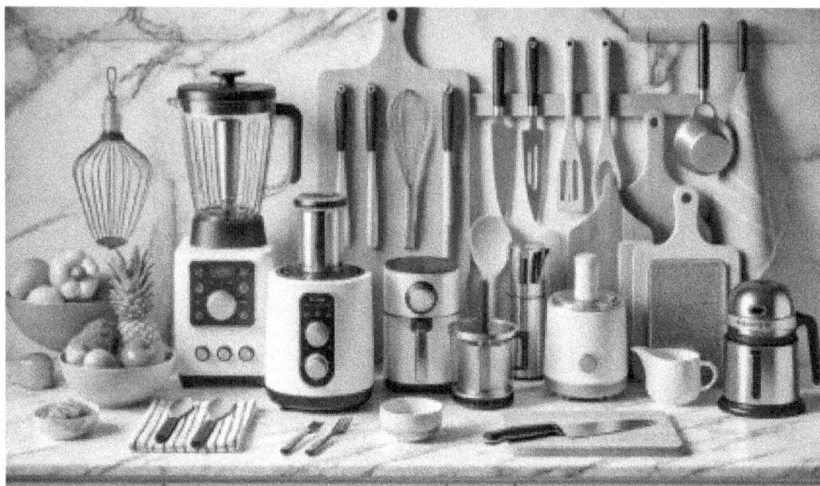

Chapter 4: Kitchen Must-Haves: Essential Tools and Appliances

Introduction: The Power of the Right Tools

Creating healthy meals becomes much easier with the right tools and equipment. You don't need a gourmet kitchen stocked with every gadget on the market, but investing in a few essential items can save time and make cooking at home more enjoyable. This chapter highlights the must-have tools for a healthy kitchen and offers recommendations for working within your budget or upgrading to premium options.

Section 1: Essential Appliances for Healthy Cooking

1. Blender or High-Speed Blender

- **Uses:** Smoothies, soups, sauces, and homemade nut butters.

- **Budget Option:** NutriBullet or Hamilton Beach Blender.

- **Premium Option:** Vitamix or Blendtec—ideal for smoothies, soups, and even doughs.

1. Air Fryer

- **Uses:** A healthier alternative to frying, perfect for crispy veggies, chicken, and more.

- **Budget Option:** GoWISE USA Air Fryer.

- **Premium Option:** Philips Premium Airfryer XXL.

1. Slow Cooker or Instant Pot

- **Uses:** Great for soups, stews, and batch-cooking beans and grains.

- **Budget Option:** Crock-Pot.

- **Premium Option:** Instant Pot Duo—it functions as a pressure cooker, slow cooker, and rice cooker all in one.

1. Food Processor

- **Uses:** Chopping vegetables, making hummus, nut butter, or pesto.

- **Budget Option:** Cuisinart Mini-Prep.

- **Premium Option:** Breville Sous Chef 16-Cup.

1. **Rice Cooker or Multicooker**

- **Uses:** Perfectly cooked rice, quinoa, or oatmeal without supervision.

- **Budget Option:** Aroma Rice Cooker.

- **Premium Option:** Zojirushi Induction Heating Rice Cooker.

Section 2: Must-Have Utensils and Tools

1. **Chef's Knife**

- **Importance:** A sharp, quality knife is essential for efficient prep.

- **Budget Option:** Victorinox Fibrox Pro Chef's Knife.

- **Premium Option:** Wüsthof or Shun Classic Chef's Knife.

1. **Cutting Boards**

- **Tip:** Use separate boards for produce and proteins to avoid cross-contamination.

- **Budget Option:** Plastic boards with non-slip edges.

- **Premium Option:** Boos Block Maple Wood Cutting Board.

1. **Measuring Cups and Spoons**

- **Why It's Essential:** Precision matters in healthy cooking and baking.

1. **Silicone Spatulas and Tongs**

- **Uses:** Stirring, flipping, and scraping without damaging non-stick surfaces.

1. **Cast Iron Skillet or Non-Stick Pan**

- **Uses:** Great for searing proteins or roasting vegetables.

- **Budget Option:** Lodge Cast Iron Skillet.

1. Baking Sheets and Parchment Paper

- **Uses:** Roasting vegetables, baking salmon, or making granola.

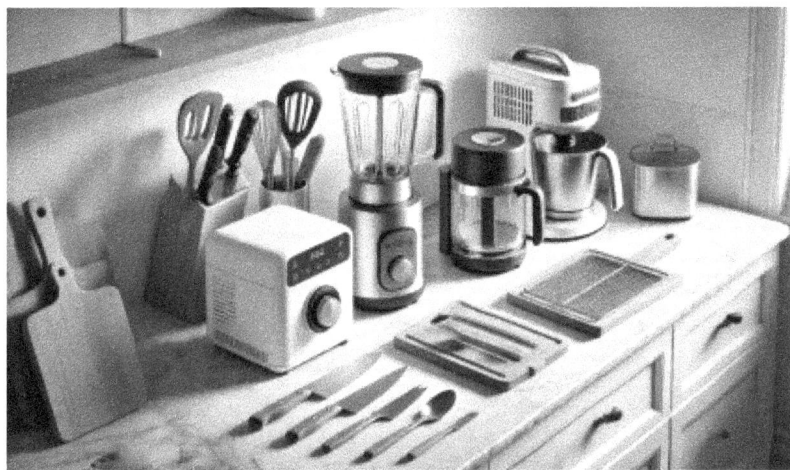

Chapter 5: Integrating What You Have: A Healthy Kitchen on a Fixed Budget

Introduction: Making the Most of Limited Resources

Creating a healthy kitchen doesn't require you to throw out everything you own or buy expensive replacements. In fact, part of the journey to healthy living is learning how to repurpose what you already have and make strategic improvements over time. This chapter will walk you through creative ways to transform your kitchen using the resources you already have, along with tips for meal planning, shopping on a budget, and repurposing pantry staples.

Section 1: Start With What's Already in Your Kitchen

Before buying anything new, it's essential to make an inventory of your current pantry, fridge, and tools. Many of the items you already own can be repurposed or modified to support healthy habits.

Inventory Checklist:

- **Dry Goods:** Grains, pasta, beans, and lentils

- **Spices and Seasonings:** Salt, pepper, herbs, spices

- **Canned Items:** Vegetables, tomatoes, beans, or broth

- **Frozen Foods:** Vegetables, fruits, or leftovers

- **Tools and Appliances:** Pots, pans, knives, storage containers

Pro Tip: Take this opportunity to declutter and organize your kitchen. Donate unopened non-perishables you don't plan to use to a local food bank.

Section 2: Adapting Pantry Staples for Healthy Meals

You don't need to buy all-new ingredients to eat healthily. Often, the items you already have can be used creatively in nutritious recipes.

Ideas for Pantry-First Recipes:

- **Chili:** Use canned beans, tomatoes, and spices to create a hearty, healthy chili.

- **Vegetable Stir-Fry:** Frozen vegetables, leftover rice, and a splash of soy sauce make for a quick meal.

- **Pasta Salad:** Combine whole wheat pasta with canned beans and chopped vegetables.

- **Smoothies:** Blend frozen fruits, oats, and any kind of milk for a quick breakfast or snack.

Section 3: Smart Shopping When You're on a Tight Budget

Shopping strategically is essential when you're working with a limited budget. Here are tips to get the most value out of your grocery trips:

1. **Make a List Based on Your Meal Plan:** Avoid impulse purchases by sticking to your list.

1. **Buy in Bulk When Possible:** Items like grains, beans, and spices are cheaper in bulk.

1. **Choose Store Brands:** Store brands often offer the same quality at a lower price.

1. **Shop Discount and Outlet Stores:** Stores like Aldi, Grocery Outlet, or local co-ops can offer great deals.

1. **Use Apps for Coupons:** Apps like Ibotta or Fetch Rewards help you save money.

Pro Tip: When possible, compare prices between local stores and online platforms like Amazon or Walmart to find the best deals.

Section 4: Stretching Your Meals With Batch Cooking and Freezing

Batch cooking is a budget-friendly way to ensure you always have healthy meals available. Cook large quantities of meals that freeze well, like soups, stews, and casseroles, and portion them into individual servings.

Examples of Batch-Friendly Meals:

- **Vegetable Soup:** Use whatever fresh or frozen vegetables you have on hand.

- **Oatmeal:** Cook a large batch of oats and refrigerate portions for quick breakfasts.

- **Chickpea Curry:** Combine canned chickpeas with curry paste and coconut milk.

- **Quinoa Bowls:** Make a base of quinoa and top with roasted vegetables and protein.

Pro Tip: Label your containers with the contents and date to make it easy to grab meals when needed.

Section 5: Making Healthy Snacks With Limited Ingredients

Buying pre-packaged healthy snacks can be expensive. Instead, use simple ingredients you already have to create your own snacks.

Easy DIY Snack Ideas:

- **Popcorn:** Air-pop kernels and season with nutritional yeast or cinnamon.

- **Trail Mix:** Combine nuts, seeds, and dried fruit.

- **Energy Bites:** Blend oats, peanut butter, and honey into bite-sized balls.

- **Fruit and Nut Butter:** Slice apples or bananas and pair with almond or peanut butter.

Pro Tip: Keep snacks pre-portioned in small containers or bags for quick grabs.

Section 6: Repurpose Leftovers and Avoid Food Waste

One of the biggest ways to save money is by repurposing leftovers into new meals. With a little creativity, yesterday's dinner can become today's lunch or even a new dish entirely.

Ways to Repurpose Leftovers:

- **Leftover Vegetables:** Add them to scrambled eggs or a frittata.

- **Cooked Grains:** Use leftover rice or quinoa to make veggie bowls.

- **Roasted Chicken:** Turn it into chicken salad or tacos.

- **Stale Bread:** Make croutons or blend it into breadcrumbs.

Section 7: Tools You Can Use Without Breaking the Bank

While it's nice to have the latest kitchen gadgets, most healthy meals can be made with just a few basic tools. If you're working with a limited budget, focus on these essentials:

- **Knife and Cutting Board:** Essential for almost every meal.

- **Non-Stick or Cast-Iron Pan:** Versatile for everything from stir-fries to pancakes.

- **Mixing Bowls:** Useful for salads, marinades, and meal prep.

- **Blender:** Perfect for smoothies, soups, and sauces.

- **Storage Containers:** Essential for storing leftovers and meal prep.

Section 8: Affordable Healthy Ingredients to Stock Up On

When building a healthy kitchen on a budget, focus on versatile, nutrient-dense foods that are affordable and long-lasting.

Affordable Ingredients to Prioritize:

- **Grains:** Oats, brown rice, and whole wheat pasta

- **Proteins:** Eggs, beans, lentils, tofu

- **Vegetables:** Frozen vegetables, carrots, onions, spinach

- **Fruits:** Bananas, apples, frozen berries

- **Healthy Fats:** Peanut butter, olive oil, avocado oil

Pro Tip: Stick with simple, unprocessed ingredients that can be used across multiple meals.

Section 9: Free and Low-Cost Resources for Healthy Eating

If you're on a tight budget, there are plenty of free or low-cost resources to help you along the way.

- **Local Food Pantries:** Many food banks offer fresh produce and pantry staples.

- **SNAP Benefits:** Check if you qualify for government assistance to help with groceries.

- **Community Gardens:** Grow your own food with access to a shared garden plot.

- **Library Cookbooks:** Borrow cookbooks focused on healthy, affordable meals.

- **YouTube Tutorials:** Channels like *Budget Bytes* offer budget-friendly recipe ideas.

Conclusion: You Can Build a Healthy Kitchen, No Matter Your Budget

Building a healthy kitchen doesn't have to be expensive. With a little creativity, smart shopping, and thoughtful meal planning, you can make the most of what you already have while gradually incorporating healthier choices. Whether you're working with a limited budget or simply looking to reduce waste, every small change you make brings you closer to a healthier lifestyle.

In the next chapter, we'll explore what it looks like to go all-in—when budget isn't a concern, and you're ready to fully invest in creating the ultimate healthy kitchen.

Section 3: Tools for Meal Prep and Storage

1. **Glass Meal Prep Containers**

- **Uses:** Storing leftovers and portioning out meals.

1. **Mason Jars**

- **Uses:** Perfect for salads, overnight oats, and homemade dressings.

1. **Reusable Silicone Bags**

- **Uses:** Storing snacks or freezing fruits and vegetables without the waste of plastic bags.

1. **Salad Spinner**

- **Uses:** Quickly dries greens to keep them crisp for salads or storage.

Section 4: Tools and Gadgets Worth the Splurge

If your budget allows for a few upgrades, these tools can make a big difference:

- **Immersion Blender:** Ideal for blending soups and sauces directly in the pot.

- **Digital Kitchen Scale:** Helps with portion control and precision in baking.

- **Electric Kettle:** A quick and easy way to boil water for tea, oatmeal, or pour-over coffee.

- **Stand Mixer:** Perfect for those who bake regularly or make homemade bread.

Section 5: How to Organize and Store Your Tools Effectively

An organized kitchen makes it easier to find what you need and encourages healthy cooking habits.

1. **Drawer Dividers:** Use dividers to keep utensils organized.

1. **Hanging Racks or Magnetic Strips:** Store knives and frequently used tools within easy reach.

1. **Lazy Susans:** Maximize space in cabinets and pantries.

1. **Over-the-Door Organizers:** Perfect for storing baking sheets, cutting boards, or spices.

1. **Labeling:** Label jars, containers, and bins for easy identification.

Section 6: Building a Healthy Kitchen on a Budget

If you're working with a limited budget, here's how to prioritize your spending:

1. **With the Essentials:** Focus on a sharp knife, cutting board, and a basic pan.

1. **Buy Secondhand:** Check thrift stores or online marketplaces for lightly used appliances.

1. **Look for Sales:** Take advantage of holiday discounts to invest in high-quality tools.

1. **DIY Storage Solutions:** Use recycled glass jars and containers for food storage.

Section 7: Resources for Finding Tools and Appliances on a Budget

- **Secondhand Stores:** Goodwill, Habitat for Humanity ReStores

- **Online Marketplaces:** Facebook Marketplace, OfferUp, Craigslist

- **Outlet Stores:** Look for kitchen tools at discount stores like TJ Maxx, Marshalls, or HomeGoods.

- **Amazon Warehouse:** Find discounted appliances and tools in Amazon's "Warehouse Deals" section.

Section 8: Maintenance and Care Tips to Make Tools Last

Caring for your tools extends their lifespan and keeps them in top shape. Here are some maintenance tips:

- **Sharpen Knives Regularly:** A dull knife is more dangerous than a sharp one.

- **Season Cast Iron Pans:** Keep them rust-free and non-stick with regular seasoning.

- **Clean Appliances Thoroughly:** Follow the manufacturer's instructions for cleaning blenders, air fryers, and slow cookers.

- **Store Tools Properly:** Use protective covers for knives and stack pans carefully to avoid scratches.

Conclusion: The Right Tools Empower a Healthy Kitchen

Having the right tools and appliances can transform your kitchen experience. You don't need every gadget under the sun, but having a few well-chosen tools makes healthy cooking more enjoyable and sustainable. Whether you're starting with the basics or investing in premium upgrades, each tool is an investment in your well-being.

In the next chapter, we'll explore the endless possibilities of building a healthy kitchen when money is no object—highlighting the tools, ingredients, and resources that can take your kitchen to the next level.

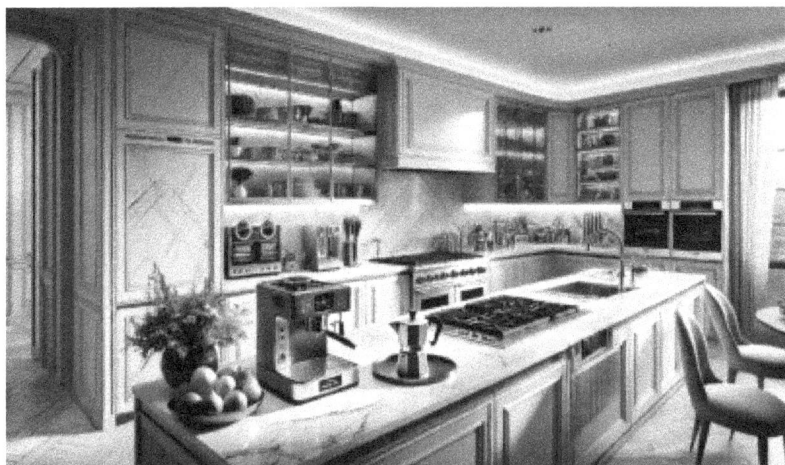

Chapter 6: All-In: What a Healthy Kitchen Looks Like When Money Is No Object

Introduction: Investing in Your Health Through Your Kitchen

When the budget is unlimited, the possibilities for creating a healthy kitchen are endless. This chapter explores what it looks like to design a high-end, functional kitchen that supports healthy eating. From top-tier appliances to premium ingredients, this is the blueprint for creating a dream kitchen that makes healthy cooking seamless and enjoyable.

Section 1: The Ultimate Healthy Kitchen Layout

The design and flow of your kitchen play a significant role in how easily you can prepare nutritious meals. Here's what an ideal layout looks like:

1. **Dedicated Prep Zone:** A large countertop with easy access to knives, cutting boards, and ingredients.

1. **Separate Stations:** A smoothie station, baking corner, and coffee or tea bar make meal prep fun and efficient.

1. **Open Shelving for Essentials:** Keep frequently used items like spices, oils, and grains visible.

1. **Pantry Walk-In:** Stock with whole foods, grains, canned goods, and specialty ingredients.

1. **Double-Sink Setup:** One sink for washing produce and another for cleaning up after meals.

1. **Custom Lighting:** Bright lighting over prep areas and softer lighting for dining spaces.

Section 2: High-End Appliances for the Ultimate Kitchen

With no financial restrictions, you can invest in state-of-the-art appliances that make healthy cooking easier and more enjoyable.

1. **Professional-Grade Blender:** Vitamix A3500 or Blendtec Pro Series for smoothies, soups, and nut butters.

1. **Air Fryer Oven:** Breville Smart Oven Air for air frying, baking, and dehydrating.

1. **Sous Vide Cooker:** Perfectly cook meats and vegetables to retain nutrients and moisture.

1. **Smart Refrigerator:** Samsung Family Hub Refrigerator with built-in cameras to track food inventory.

1. **Steam Oven:** Miele Steam Oven for healthy, oil-free cooking.

1. **Induction Cooktop:** Faster, more energy-efficient cooking with precise temperature control.

Section 3: Premium Ingredients to Elevate Your Healthy Kitchen

When money is no object, you can afford to stock your kitchen with the finest ingredients for health and flavor.

- **Organic, Locally-Sourced Produce:** Prioritize seasonal fruits and vegetables from farmers' markets or local farms.

- **Grass-Fed and Organic Meats:** Look for hormone-free, pasture-raised options.

- **Wild-Caught Seafood:** Choose high-quality fish like salmon, cod, and shellfish.

- **Artisanal Whole Grains:** Farro, freekeh, and heirloom quinoa.

- **Premium Oils:** Extra virgin olive oil, walnut oil, and avocado oil.

- **Specialty Superfoods:** Spirulina, matcha, maca powder, and acai.

Section 4: Gourmet Kitchen Tools Worth the Investment

Here are high-end tools that bring luxury and function to your kitchen:

1. **Precision Knife Set:** Japanese Damascus steel knives for ultimate sharpness and durability.

1. **Custom Cutting Boards:** Walnut or teak boards that are both functional and beautiful.

1. **Smart Kitchen Scale:** Track macros and portion sizes with Bluetooth-connected scales.

1. **Espresso Machine:** A high-quality espresso machine for homemade lattes and specialty drinks.

1. **Copper Cookware Set:** Handcrafted copper pots and pans for excellent heat conductivity.

Section 5: Specialty Equipment for Advanced Healthy Cooking

For those who enjoy experimenting with recipes, these specialized tools open new culinary possibilities:

1. **Dehydrator:** Make your own dried fruits, vegetable chips, or jerky.

1. **Fermentation Kit:** Brew kombucha, pickle vegetables, or make homemade yogurt.

1. **Cold-Pressed Juicer:** Extract nutrient-dense juices with minimal oxidation.

1. **Tandoor Oven:** For traditional, healthy flatbreads and roasted dishes.

Section 6: Design Features to Enhance Your Kitchen Experience

A beautiful and well-designed kitchen encourages you to spend more time preparing healthy meals.

- **Marble or Quartz Countertops:** Durable and easy to clean.

- **Custom Spice Drawers:** Organize herbs and spices for easy access.

- **Built-In Herb Garden:** Grow fresh basil, mint, or parsley indoors.

- **Wine Fridge:** Store organic wines or kombucha at optimal temperatures.

- **Built-In Compost System:** Minimize food waste while supporting sustainable practices.

Section 7: Hiring Experts to Support Your Health Journey

With the resources to invest in your health, you can bring in experts to assist with meal planning and preparation.

- **Nutritionist or Dietitian:** Create a personalized meal plan tailored to your needs.

- **Private Chef:** Enjoy custom-prepared healthy meals at home.

- **Meal Prep Services:** Have healthy meals delivered or prepared in advance.

- **Kitchen Designer:** Optimize your kitchen's functionality and aesthetics.

- **Personal Trainer:** Combine healthy eating with a tailored fitness program.

Section 8: The Art of Hosting Healthy Gatherings

A luxurious kitchen also becomes a space to share your healthy lifestyle with friends and family. Hosting gatherings centered around nutritious meals can inspire others to embrace healthier choices.

Ideas for Healthy Gatherings:

- **Smoothie Bar Brunch:** Let guests create their own smoothies with a variety of toppings.

- **Gourmet Salad Party:** Offer a spread of greens, vegetables, proteins, and dressings.

- **Plant-Based Dinner:** Serve creative vegan dishes that appeal to all tastes.

- **Cooking Classes:** Hire a chef to teach healthy cooking techniques.

Section 9: Resources for Designing and Stocking a Dream Kitchen

Here are some resources to help you create the ultimate healthy kitchen:

- **Design Inspiration:** Websites like Houzz or Pinterest for kitchen ideas.

- **Luxury Appliance Stores:** Sub-Zero, Wolf, and Miele showrooms.

- **Specialty Grocers:** Whole Foods, Erewhon, or local co-ops for premium ingredients.

- **Farmers' Markets Finder:** Use LocalHarvest.org to find markets near you.

- **Kitchen Designers:** Consider professionals from companies like Poggenpohl or Bulthaup.

Section 10: Balancing Luxury with Sustainability

Even in a high-end kitchen, sustainability matters. Here are ways to keep your dream kitchen environmentally friendly:

1. **Compost Your Food Scraps:** Use a built-in compost bin or countertop system.

1. **Choose Energy-Efficient Appliances:** Look for ENERGY STAR ratings.

1. **Support Local Farms:** Reduce your carbon footprint by buying locally.

1. **Minimize Plastic Use:** Opt for glass or metal storage containers.

1. **Grow Your Own Food:** Use a garden wall or hydroponic system to grow herbs and vegetables.

Conclusion: Embracing the Power of Possibility

Building the ultimate healthy kitchen allows you to fully invest in your health and well-being. With premium tools, appliances, and ingredients at your disposal, cooking becomes not just a task but an experience. Whether you're hosting healthy gatherings, working with a private chef, or simply enjoying the beauty of your space, every element contributes to a lifestyle that prioritizes nourishment, joy, and sustainability.

In the next chapter, we'll explore how to sustain these changes and build habits that stick, ensuring that your healthy kitchen remains a source of inspiration for years to come.

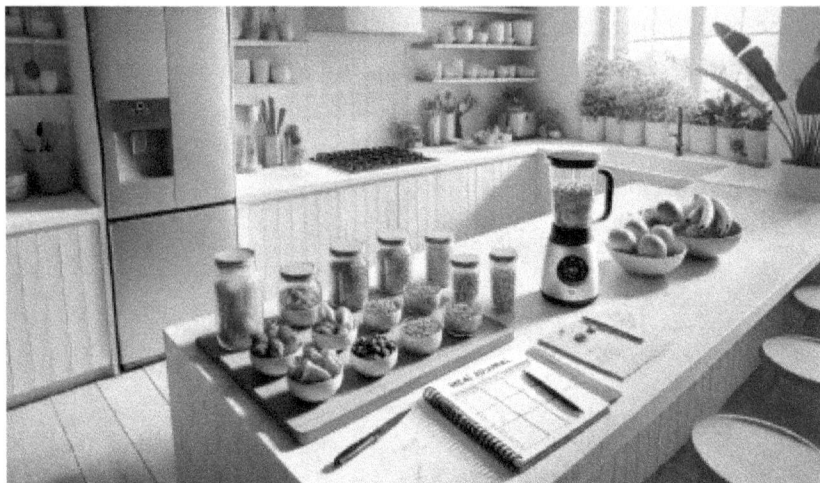

Chapter 7: Making the Shift Sustainable – Staying on Track Long-Term

Sustaining a healthy lifestyle isn't just possible—it's achievable with the right tools, mindset, and strategies. This chapter will equip you with **creative, actionable ideas** that help keep you on track, even when life gets busy, cravings hit, or motivation dips. Long-term success isn't about perfection—it's about **consistency, preparation, and enjoyment.** Below, you'll find **loads of practical advice and shortcuts** to make healthy living sustainable.

1. Managing Cravings and Occasional Indulgences Without Guilt

- **Don't Ban Your Favorite Foods Entirely:** Instead, find healthier versions of your go-to indulgences. Swap fried snacks for **air-fried alternatives** or try **dark chocolate** instead of milk chocolate.

- **Portion Control Hack:** Pre-portion indulgent foods (like chips or cookies) into **small bags or containers** to avoid overindulging.

- **Fruit First Strategy:** Keep **ready-to-eat fruits** (like grapes, berries, or sliced apples) at eye level in your fridge or on the counter. When cravings strike, you're more likely to grab what's convenient and visible.

- **"Indulgence Day" Strategy:** Set aside one meal or treat a week for indulgence without guilt. Enjoy it fully, knowing it's part of your healthy plan.

2. Developing Healthy Habits That Stick Beyond the Kitchen

- **Visual Cues:** Keep reminders of your goals visible—whether it's a **whiteboard meal plan** in the kitchen or a list of healthy habits on your fridge.

- **Habit Stacking:** Build new healthy habits onto existing routines. For example, while you wait for your coffee to brew, use that time to prep a smoothie or pack a healthy snack for later.

- **Make Hydration Automatic:** Place **water bottles or fruit-infused pitchers** around the house to encourage hydration throughout the day.

- **Automate Healthy Eating:** Use meal-prepping shortcuts like making **double portions of dinner** and freezing half for later.

- **Daily Movement**: Incorporate small moments of physical activity throughout your day. Even 10-minute walks or stretching between tasks can add up to significant health benefits over time.

3. Tracking Progress Without Obsessing Over Perfection

- **Non-Scale Victories:** Track progress beyond the scale—like better energy, clearer skin, or improved sleep.

- **Journaling for Reflection:** Keep a simple journal to note how you feel after meals or workouts to connect with the changes in your body.

- **Set Milestones, Not Deadlines:** Focus on small wins, such as preparing three healthy meals a week or drinking more water consistently.

- **Use Technology Wisely:** Try apps that remind you to drink water, log meals, or track steps, but don't let perfectionism take over. Healthy living is a **lifelong journey**, not a race.

4. Encouraging Family and Friends to Join the Journey

- **Family Meals as a Celebration:** Cook meals together and create traditions around healthy food—like a **smoothie bar for breakfast** or "Meatless Mondays."

- **Involve Kids in the Kitchen:** Let children pick a healthy recipe or help with simple tasks like stirring or setting the table. This teaches them the importance of food and health.

- **Invite Accountability:** Create **group challenges** with family or friends—like weekly steps challenges or recipe swaps. Sharing the journey keeps it fun and builds accountability.

- **Lead by Example:** When family and friends see you enjoying healthy meals and thriving, they'll be inspired to join you naturally.

5. Creative Shortcuts and Ideas to Sustain Healthy Habits

- **Repurpose Leftovers:** Transform last night's roast chicken into **fajitas or stir-fry.** Turn extra veggies into an **omelet** the next day.

- **Smoothie Prep Hack:** Pre-portion frozen smoothie ingredients into zip-lock bags for quick blending on busy mornings.

- **Portable Snacks:** Keep **pre-portioned nuts, trail mix, or grapes** in bags for quick, healthy snacks on the go.

- **Use Kitchen Gadgets to Save Time:** Invest in tools like an **instant pot, air fryer, or food processor** to make meal prep faster and easier.

- **Batch-Cook Proteins:** Grill or bake a variety of proteins (like chicken, salmon, or tofu) in one session and store them for easy meals throughout the week.

- **Freezer Friendly Meals:** Double recipes like soups, stews, and casseroles to freeze for busy days. Label containers with dates to keep track.

- **Grocery List Hack:** Use a **master grocery list** with healthy staples and keep it on your phone for easy access when shopping.

6. Is Long-Term Success Possible? Yes! Here's How to Stay Motivated

- **Celebrate Your Wins:** Take time to celebrate every milestone, no matter how small. Whether it's prepping a week's worth of meals or drinking more water, every effort matters.

- **Make Health Enjoyable:** Find joy in cooking, trying new recipes, or exercising. When it feels fun, it's easier to stay motivated.

- **Focus on the Process, Not Perfection:** Remember that setbacks are part of the journey. The key is to keep moving forward, no matter how small the steps.

- **Surround Yourself with Support:** Build a community of like-minded people who encourage you. Join online groups, find a workout buddy, or share your journey with family and friends.

- **Use Visual Reminders of Your Why:** Place inspiring quotes or pictures where you can see them daily. Staying connected to your "why" will keep you grounded on tough days.

Conclusion: The Journey Continues

Sustaining healthy habits isn't about doing everything perfectly—it's about making **consistent, intentional choices** every day. With the tools, strategies, and insights from this book, you are well-equipped to build a lifestyle that supports your goals. Remember, this is a lifelong journey, and **every small effort counts**.

Celebrate your progress, embrace the joy of healthy living, and continue to build on what you've learned. Your kitchen is now a space for growth, nourishment, and transformation—**a place where health begins and thrives.** You have what it takes to live the vibrant, healthy life you envision. Now, step forward and make it happen!

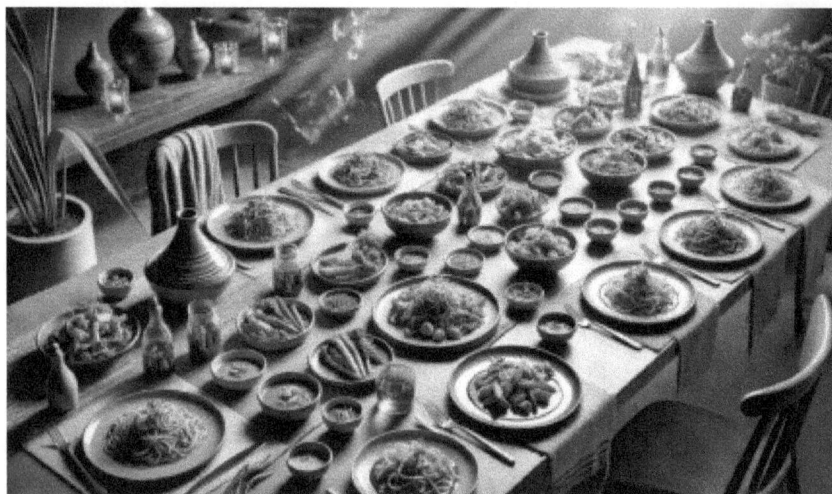

Part 2 Introduction: Now the Fun Begins—Cooking with Heart and Purpose

Congratulations! You've taken the first and most important step toward a healthier lifestyle by transforming your kitchen. With the tools, ingredients, and habits you've cultivated in Part One, you've laid a solid foundation for success. You now have everything you need to sustain a lifestyle of wellness and joy, but the journey doesn't stop here. This is where it truly begins.

A healthy kitchen is not just about what's in your pantry or refrigerator—it's about what you create with those ingredients. It's about crafting meals that nourish both body and soul, meals that align with your health goals without compromising taste, satisfaction, or budget. This next section is designed to take you from planning and preparing to *doing*—bringing your healthy kitchen to life with recipes that are as delightful to eat as they are to make.

The Purpose of This Section: Putting Tools into Practice

In the following chapters, you'll find carefully crafted recipes that reflect the principles of a healthy lifestyle. Each recipe is built around whole foods, balanced nutrition, and bold flavors. But there's more—these dishes aren't just good for you; they're also designed to feel like a treat. Healthy doesn't mean boring or restrictive. Whether it's a refreshing salad, a hearty soup, a nourishing entrée, or a decadent dessert, these recipes will help you enjoy eating well.

What makes these recipes unique is that they are achievable, regardless of budget. Many people assume that healthy cooking is expensive or time-consuming, but these recipes are here to prove otherwise. They leverage affordable ingredients and simple techniques to create restaurant-quality dishes without breaking your diet or your wallet.

A Balanced Approach: Exquisite Yet Practical Recipes

One of the goals of this section is to offer variety and versatility. Everyone has their own preferences, dietary needs, and time constraints, so you'll find options that fit into different lifestyles. Whether you prefer plant-based meals, enjoy hearty proteins, or need quick snacks for busy days, there's something for everyone. Each section is filled with easy-to-follow instructions to make cooking accessible, even for beginners.

We've also divided the recipes into six essential categories:

1. **Salads:** Light yet filling, packed with vibrant ingredients and balanced dressings.

1. **Soups:** Warm and nourishing bowls that are perfect for any season.

1. **Entrées:** Hearty meals that keep you satisfied while staying on track.

1. **Desserts:** Guilt-free sweets that feel indulgent but fit into your healthy lifestyle.

1. **Snacks:** On-the-go options to fuel your day between meals.

1. **Smoothies:** Power-packed drinks that make breakfast or post-workout fuel effortless.

What to Expect: Detailed, Step-by-Step Instructions

Unlike typical cookbooks that simply list ingredients and instructions, we've gone the extra mile to provide clear, detailed directions. Every recipe includes step-by-step guidance so you'll never feel lost. This isn't about throwing ingredients together—it's about building flavor, enjoying the process, and creating something you're proud to eat.

You'll also find tips for ingredient substitutions, meal prepping, and pairing dishes together for complete meals. These recipes reflect the idea that food can be healthy, affordable, and delicious, all at once. Whether you're cooking for yourself or hosting friends and family, these meals are designed to impress.

Cooking with Heart: Creating Meals with Meaning

Beyond nutrition, these recipes aim to bring joy and mindfulness to your time in the kitchen. Cooking isn't just about following instructions—it's about connecting with the food you eat, appreciating the process, and sharing that experience with others. Every meal is an opportunity to honor the effort you've put into building your healthy kitchen.

We encourage you to be creative. Use these recipes as a guide, but feel free to experiment, swap ingredients, and make them your own. A healthy kitchen isn't about rigid rules—it's about finding what works for you and embracing the journey.

Looking Forward: Let's Get Cooking!

Now it's time to dive in and bring everything you've learned to life. We'll start with salads—light, refreshing, and perfect for any time of day. From there, we'll explore soups, entrées, desserts, snacks, and smoothies, each with its own chapter. Whether you're making a quick lunch or preparing a feast, these recipes will help you enjoy the process and the results.

So, grab your favorite fork, turn on some music, and let's get cooking. Your healthy kitchen is ready to shine, and we can't wait to see what you create.

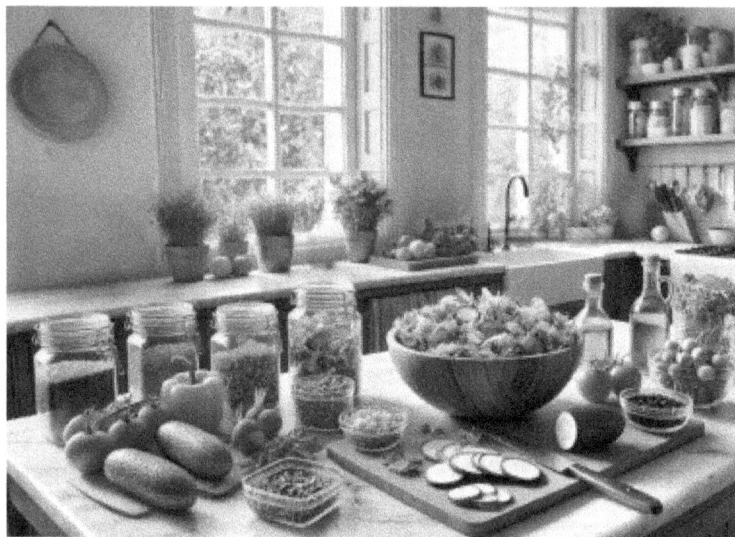

Part 2: Chapter 1: Vibrant and Satisfying Salads

Introduction to Salads

Salads often get a bad reputation for being bland or unsatisfying, but when done right, they can be the star of the table. The following five salads combine fresh ingredients, bold dressings, and nutrient-dense components that will leave you feeling full and energized. Each salad can serve as a light meal on its own or as a complement to an entrée.

Recipe 1: Mediterranean Chickpea Salad

Serves: 4 | **Prep Time:** 20 minutes
Ingredients:

- 1 can (15 oz) chickpeas, drained and rinsed

- 1 cucumber, diced

- 1-pint cherry tomatoes, halved

- 1 red bell pepper, diced

- ½ red onion, thinly sliced

- ¼ cup Kalamata olives, pitted and halved

- ½ cup feta cheese, crumbled

- ¼ cup fresh parsley, chopped

- 2 tbsp olive oil

- 1 tbsp red wine vinegar

- 1 tsp dried oregano

- Salt and pepper to taste

Instructions:

1. In a large bowl, combine the chickpeas, cucumber, tomatoes, bell pepper, red onion, and olives.

1. In a small bowl, whisk together the olive oil, red wine vinegar, oregano, salt, and pepper.

1. Pour the dressing over the salad and toss to combine.

1. Gently fold in the feta cheese and parsley.

1. Serve immediately or refrigerate for up to 3 days for the flavors to meld.

Pro Tip: Add grilled chicken or tuna for extra protein.

Recipe 2: Quinoa and Roasted Vegetable Salad

Serves: 4 | Prep Time: 15 minutes | Cook Time: 25 minutes

Ingredients:

- 1 cup of quinoa, rinsed

- 2 cups of water or vegetable broth

- 1 zucchini, sliced

- 1 bell pepper (any color), sliced

- 1 red onion, cut into wedges

- 1 cup cherry tomatoes, halved

- 2 tbsp olive oil

- ½ tsp garlic powder

- Salt and pepper to taste

- ½ cup crumbled goat cheese (optional)

- ¼ cup basil, chopped

Instructions:

1. Preheat the oven to 400°F (200°C).

1. Toss the zucchini, bell pepper, red onion, and cherry tomatoes with olive oil, garlic powder, salt, and pepper. Spread on a baking sheet and roast for 20-25 minutes.

1. While the vegetables roast, bring the quinoa and water (or broth) to a boil. Reduce heat, cover, and simmer for 15 minutes or until the quinoa is cooked and fluffy.

1. Combine the quinoa and roasted vegetables in a large bowl.

1. Fold in the goat cheese (if using) and chopped basil.

1. Serve warm or chilled.

Recipe 3: Kale Caesar Salad with Crispy Chickpeas

Serves: 4 | **Prep Time:** 20 minutes
Ingredients:

- 1 bunch kale, stems removed, and leaves torn

- 1 can (15 oz) chickpeas, drained and rinsed

- 2 tbsp olive oil

- 1 tsp smoked paprika

- ½ cup grated Parmesan cheese

- ¼ cup Caesar dressing (store-bought or homemade)

- Juice of ½ lemon

Instructions:

1. Preheat the oven to 375°F (190°C). Toss the chickpeas with olive oil and smoked paprika and spread them on a baking sheet. Roast for 20 minutes until crispy.

1. Massage the kale with a bit of olive oil and lemon juice for 2-3 minutes to soften the leaves.

1. Add the Parmesan cheese and Caesar dressing to the kale, and toss to coat evenly.

1. Top with crispy chickpeas. Serve immediately.

Pro Tip: Add grilled shrimp or salmon for a heartier version.

Recipe 4: Strawberry Spinach Salad with Poppy Seed Dressing

Serves: 4 | **Prep Time:** 15 minutes
Ingredients:

- 6 cups baby spinach

- 1 cup strawberries, sliced

- ¼ red onion, thinly sliced

- ½ cup crumbled feta or goat cheese

- ¼ cup slivered almonds, toasted

- ¼ cup balsamic glaze

For the Dressing:

- 3 tbsp olive oil

- 2 tbsp white vinegar

- 1 tbsp honey

- 1 tsp poppy seeds

- Pinch of salt

Instructions:

1. In a large bowl, combine the spinach, strawberries, red onion, and almonds.

1. In a small bowl, whisk together the dressing ingredients.

1. Drizzle the dressing over the salad and toss gently.

1. Top with crumbled feta or goat cheese.

1. Drizzle with balsamic glaze just before serving.

Pro Tip: Swap the strawberries for blueberries or peaches based on the season.

Recipe 5: Asian Cabbage Salad with Sesame Ginger Dressing

Serves: 4 | **Prep Time:** 20 minutes

Ingredients:

- 4 cups shredded green or Napa cabbage

- 2 carrots, julienned

- 1 red bell pepper, thinly sliced

- 1 cucumber, sliced into half moons

- ¼ cup chopped cilantro

- 2 tbsp sesame seeds, toasted

For the Dressing:

- 3 tbsp sesame oil

- 2 tbsp rice vinegar

- 1 tbsp soy sauce or tamari

- 1 tbsp honey or maple syrup

- 1 tsp grated ginger

- 1 garlic clove, minced

Instructions:

1. In a large bowl, combine the cabbage, carrots, bell pepper, cucumber, and cilantro.

1. In a small bowl, whisk together the dressing ingredients.

1. Pour the dressing over the salad and toss to combine.

1. Sprinkle with toasted sesame seeds before serving.

Pro Tip: Add grilled tofu or chicken to turn this into a complete meal.

Conclusion: Salads That Satisfy

These salads go beyond the basics, proving that healthy eating doesn't have to be boring or bland. From Mediterranean flavors to Asian-inspired creations, each dish is packed with color, nutrition, and taste. These recipes can serve as light meals, starters, or sides—perfect for any occasion.

Up next: **Soups**—warm, nourishing bowls that will keep you cozy and full, no matter the season.

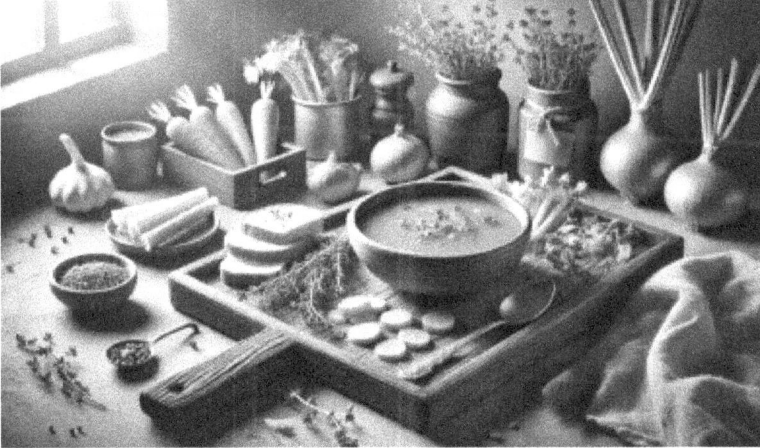

Part 2: Chapter 2: Warm and Nourishing Soups

Introduction to Soups

Soups are a perfect way to nourish your body while enjoying a comforting meal. Whether you're in the mood for something light or need a hearty bowl to fill you up, these soups have you covered. They're packed with vegetables, proteins, and bold flavors to make sure every spoonful counts. Each recipe balances taste and nutrition without straining your budget.

Recipe 1: Sweet Potato and Carrot Soup with Ginger and Curry

Serves: 6 | Prep Time: 15 minutes | Cook Time: 30 minutes
Ingredients:

- 2 tbsp olive oil

- 1 onion, chopped

- 2 garlic cloves, minced

- 1-inch piece ginger, grated

- 3 large carrots, peeled and sliced

- 2 sweet potatoes, peeled and cubed

- 1 tsp curry powder

- ½ tsp cumin

- 4 cups vegetable broth

- 1 can (14 oz) coconut milk

- Salt and pepper to taste

- Fresh cilantro for garnish

Instructions:

1. Heat the olive oil in a large pot over medium heat. Add the onion, garlic, and ginger, sautéing for 5-7 minutes until softened and fragrant.

1. Stir in the carrots and sweet potatoes, cooking for another 5 minutes.

1. Add the curry powder, cumin, salt, and pepper. Stir well to coat the vegetables with spices.

1. Pour in the vegetable broth, bring to a boil, and reduce to a simmer. Cook for 20-25 minutes until the vegetables are tender.

1. Use an immersion blender to puree the soup until smooth. Stir in the coconut milk for extra creaminess.

1. Adjust seasoning if needed. Serve hot, garnished with fresh cilantro.

Conclusion: A Unique Addition to the Soup Chapter

This Sweet Potato and Carrot Soup with Ginger and Curry offers a new, flavorful option that complements the other soups without repeating the lentil-based ingredients from the entrée chapter. It provides warmth, richness, and vibrant colors, making it perfect for both cozy nights and light lunches.

Recipe 2: Creamy Butternut Squash Soup
Serves: 4 | **Prep Time:** 15 minutes | **Cook Time:** 30 minutes
Ingredients:

- 1 butternut squash, peeled and cubed

- 2 tbsp olive oil

- 1 onion, chopped

- 2 garlic cloves, minced

- 4 cups vegetable broth

- ½ tsp cinnamon

- ½ tsp nutmeg

- Salt and pepper to taste

- ½ cup coconut milk (optional)

- Pumpkin seeds for garnish

Instructions:

1. Heat the olive oil in a large pot. Add the onion and garlic, sautéing until translucent.

1. Add the cubed squash, broth, cinnamon, nutmeg, salt, and pepper.

1. Bring to a boil, then reduce heat and simmer for 25 minutes, until the squash is tender.

1. Use an immersion blender to puree the soup until smooth.

1. Stir in the coconut milk for extra creaminess (optional).

1. Serve topped with pumpkin seeds for crunch.

Recipe 3: Chicken and Wild Rice Soup

Serves: 6 | **Prep Time:** 20 minutes | **Cook Time:** 40 minutes
Ingredients:

- 2 tbsp butter or olive oil

- 1 onion, chopped

- 2 garlic cloves, minced

- 2 carrots, diced

- 2 celery stalks, diced

- ½ cup wild rice, rinsed

- 6 cups chicken broth

- 2 cups shredded cooked chicken

- 1 tsp thyme

- 1 tsp rosemary

- Salt and pepper to taste

- ½ cup milk or cream (optional)

Instructions:

1. Melt the butter or heat the olive oil in a large pot. Add the onion, garlic, carrots, and celery. Sauté for 5-7 minutes.

1. Add wild rice, broth, thyme, rosemary, salt, and pepper. Bring to a boil.

1. Reduce heat and simmer for 30-35 minutes, until the rice is tender.

1. Stir in the chicken for the last 5 minutes of cooking.

1. Add milk or cream if using for a richer texture.

Recipe 4: Classic Minestrone Soup

Serves: 6 | **Prep Time:** 20 minutes | **Cook Time:** 30 minutes
Ingredients:

- 2 tbsp olive oil

- 1 onion, chopped

- 3 garlic cloves, minced

- 2 carrots, diced

- 2 celery stalks, diced

- 1 zucchini, chopped

- 1 can (15 oz) diced tomatoes

- 1 can (15 oz) kidney beans, drained and rinsed

- 6 cups of vegetable broth

- 1 cup small pasta (like ditalini or elbow)

- 1 tsp oregano

- Salt and pepper to taste

- 2 cups spinach or kale

Instructions:

1. Heat the olive oil in a large pot. Add the onion, garlic, carrots, and celery. Sauté for 5-7 minutes until softened.

1. Stir in the zucchini, tomatoes, beans, broth, oregano, salt, and pepper.

1. Bring to a boil, then add the pasta. Simmer until the pasta is cooked, about 10 minutes.

1. Stir in the spinach or kale during the last 2 minutes.

1. Serve hot with crusty bread.

Recipe 5: Spicy Black Bean Soup

Serves: 4 | **Prep Time:** 10 minutes | **Cook Time:** 25 minutes
Ingredients:

- 2 tbsp olive oil

- 1 onion, chopped

- 2 garlic cloves, minced

- 1 red bell pepper, diced

- 2 cans (15 oz each) black beans, drained and rinsed

- 4 cups vegetable broth

- 1 tsp cumin

- 1 tsp chili powder

- Salt and pepper to taste

- ½ lime, juiced

- Fresh cilantro for garnish

Instructions:

1. Heat the olive oil in a pot. Add the onion, garlic, and bell pepper, and sauté for 5 minutes.

1. Stir in the black beans, broth, cumin, chili powder, salt, and pepper.

1. Bring to a boil, then reduce heat and simmer for 20 minutes.

1. Use an immersion blender to puree part of the soup, leaving some texture.

1. Stir in the lime juice and garnish with cilantro before serving.

Conclusion: Soups That Warm the Soul

These soups are perfect for meal prep, easy to store, and nourishing for both body and soul. Whether you want a creamy, comforting bowl or a broth-based soup packed with vegetables, these recipes cover every craving. Enjoy them on cold nights or when you need a quick, healthy meal.

Up next: **Entrées**—hearty dishes that will leave you full, satisfied, and energized to tackle your day.

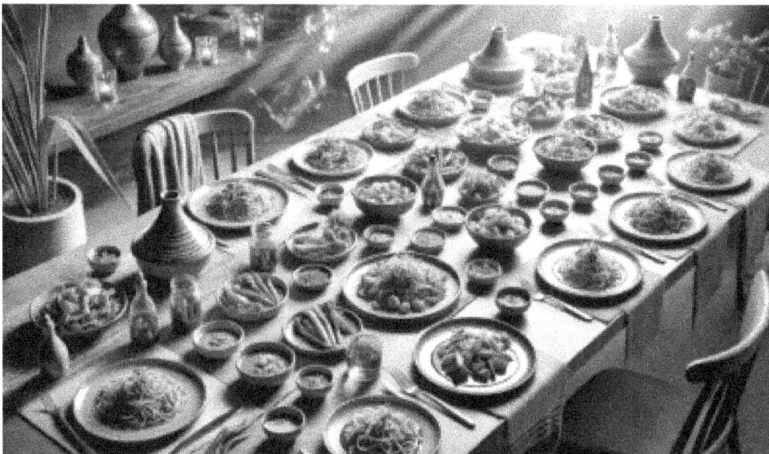

Part 2: Chapter 3: Hearty Entrées from Around the World

Introduction: A Celebration of Culinary Diversity

America is a melting pot of culinary richness, with flavors, techniques, and ingredients drawn from cultures across the globe. Food connects people, telling the stories of heritage, tradition, and identity. In this chapter, we've curated a collection of entrées that celebrate this diversity, offering dishes from African, Italian, Mexican, Asian, and Indian cuisines, among others.

Each recipe has been adapted to keep it both flavorful and nourishing, without compromising cultural authenticity. Whether you're craving bold spices, savory comfort, or vibrant flavors, these dishes bring the world to your kitchen table.

African Cuisine

Recipe 1: West African Peanut Butter Stew (Maafe)
  Serves: 6 | **Prep Time:** 15 minutes | **Cook Time:** 40 minutes
  Ingredients:

- 2 tbsp olive oil

- 1 onion, chopped

- 2 garlic cloves, minced

- 1-inch piece ginger, grated

- 1 lb chicken thighs, cut into bite-sized pieces (optional)

- 1 sweet potato, peeled and cubed

- 1 red bell pepper, diced

- 2 tbsp tomato paste

- 1 can (15 oz) diced tomatoes

- 4 cups chicken or vegetable broth

- ½ cup natural peanut butter

- 1 tsp cayenne pepper (optional)

- Salt and pepper to taste

- Fresh cilantro for garnish

Instructions:

1. Heat olive oil in a large pot over medium heat. Add onion, garlic, and ginger, and sauté until fragrant, about 5 minutes.

1. Add the chicken (if using) and cook until browned on all sides.

1. Stir in the sweet potato, bell pepper, tomato paste, and diced tomatoes. Cook for 5 minutes.

1. Pour in the broth, bring to a boil, and reduce to a simmer. Cook for 25-30 minutes, until the vegetables are tender.

1. Stir in the peanut butter until fully incorporated. Season with cayenne, salt, and pepper.

1. Serve hot, garnished with cilantro.

Recipe 2: North African Moroccan Tagine with Chickpeas and Apricots

Serves: 6 | **Prep Time:** 20 minutes | **Cook Time:** 1 hour
Ingredients:

- 2 tbsp olive oil

- 1 onion, chopped

- 3 garlic cloves, minced

- 1 tsp ground cumin

- 1 tsp cinnamon

- 1 tsp turmeric

- 2 cups of vegetable broth

- 1 can (15 oz) chickpeas, drained and rinsed

- 1 cup dried apricots, halved

- 1 zucchini, sliced

- 1 carrot, sliced

- Salt and pepper to taste

- ½ cup fresh parsley, chopped

Instructions:

1. Heat olive oil in a tagine or large pot. Add onions and garlic, and sauté until soft.

1. Stir in the cumin, cinnamon, and turmeric, and cook for 1-2 minutes until fragrant.

1. Add chickpeas, apricots, zucchini, and carrot. Pour in the broth and bring to a simmer.

1. Cover and cook on low heat for 45 minutes to 1 hour.

1. Season with salt and pepper, and garnish with fresh parsley.

Italian Cuisine

Recipe 3: Classic Chicken Piccata

Serves: 4 | **Prep Time:** 15 minutes | **Cook Time:** 20 minutes

Ingredients:

- 2 boneless, skinless chicken breasts, halved lengthwise

- Salt and pepper to taste

- ½ cup whole wheat flour

- 2 tbsp olive oil

- 2 tbsp butter

- 3 garlic cloves, minced

- ½ cup chicken broth

- ¼ cup fresh lemon juice

- 2 tbsp capers

- Fresh parsley for garnish

Instructions:

1. Season the chicken with salt and pepper, and dredge in flour, shaking off the excess.

1. Heat olive oil in a skillet over medium heat. Cook the chicken for 3-4 minutes on each side until golden brown. Set aside.

1. Add butter and garlic to the pan, and sauté for 1 minute.

1. Stir in the broth, lemon juice, and capers. Simmer for 2-3 minutes.

1. Return the chicken to the pan and spoon the sauce over it.

1. Serve with pasta or roasted vegetables, garnished with parsley.

Recipe 4: Vegetable and Quinoa Stuffed Peppers
Serves: 4 | **Prep Time:** 15 minutes | **Cook Time:** 30 minutes
Ingredients:

- 4 bell peppers, halved and seeds removed

- 1 cup cooked quinoa

- 1 zucchini, diced

- 1 cup of diced tomatoes

- ½ cup shredded mozzarella cheese

- 1 tsp Italian seasoning

- Salt and pepper to taste

Instructions:

1. Preheat the oven to 375°F (190°C).

1. In a bowl, mix the quinoa, zucchini, tomatoes, cheese, Italian seasoning, salt, and pepper.

1. Stuff the mixture into the halved bell peppers.

1. Place the peppers on a baking sheet and bake for 30 minutes until tender.

1. Serve warm.

Mexican Cuisine

Recipe 5: Chicken Enchiladas with Green Sauce
Serves: 4 | **Prep Time:** 20 minutes | **Cook Time:** 30 minutes
Ingredients:

- 8 small corn tortillas

- 2 cups of shredded chicken

- 1 cup shredded cheese (cheddar or Monterey Jack)

- 1 can (15 oz) green enchilada sauce

- 1 onion, diced

- Fresh cilantro for garnish

Instructions:

1. Preheat the oven to 350°F (175°C).

1. Fill each tortilla with chicken, cheese, and onions, and roll them tightly.

1. Place the enchiladas seam-side down in a baking dish. Pour the enchilada sauce over the top.

1. Sprinkle with remaining cheese.

1. Bake for 25-30 minutes until bubbly. Garnish with cilantro.

Recipe 6: Vegetable Tacos with Avocado Crema
Serves: 4 | **Prep Time:** 15 minutes | **Cook Time:** 10 minutes
Ingredients:

- 8 small corn tortillas

- 1 zucchini, sliced

- 1 bell pepper, sliced

- 1 red onion, sliced

- 2 tbsp olive oil

- Salt and pepper to taste

- 1 avocado, mashed

- 2 tbsp lime juice

- 2 tbsp plain Greek yogurt

Instructions:

1. Heat olive oil in a pan. Sauté the vegetables with salt and pepper until soft.

1. Mix the mashed avocado, lime juice, and yogurt to make the crema.

1. Assemble the tacos with the sautéed vegetables and drizzle with avocado crema.

Asian Cuisine

Recipe 7: Teriyaki Salmon with Steamed Vegetables
Serves: 4 | **Prep Time:** 10 minutes | **Cook Time:** 20 minutes
Ingredients:

- 4 salmon fillets

- ¼ cup soy sauce or tamari

- 2 tbsp honey

- 2 garlic cloves, minced

- Steamed broccoli and carrots

Instructions:

1. Mix soy sauce, honey, and garlic. Marinate the salmon for 10 minutes.

1. Bake the salmon at 375°F (190°C) for 15-20 minutes.

1. Serve with steamed vegetables.

Recipe 8: Stir-Fried Tofu with Vegetables
Serves: 4 | **Prep Time:** 15 minutes | **Cook Time:** 10 minutes
Ingredients:

- 1 block firm tofu, cubed

- 2 tbsp soy sauce

- 1 tsp sesame oil

- 1 red bell pepper, sliced

- 1 zucchini, sliced

Instructions:

1. Stir-fry the tofu until golden brown.

1. Add vegetables and soy sauce. Cook for 5 minutes.

French Cuisine

Recipe 17: Coq au Vin (Chicken in Red Wine)
Serves: 4 | **Prep Time:** 30 minutes | **Cook Time:** 1 hour 30 minutes
Ingredients:

- 1 whole chicken, cut into pieces

- 4 strips of bacon, chopped

- 1 onion, diced

- 3 garlic cloves, minced

- 2 cups of red wine

- 2 cups of chicken broth

- 2 carrots, sliced

- 1 tsp thyme

- 1 bay leaf

- Salt and pepper to taste

Instructions:

1. Cook the bacon in a pot until it is crispy. Remove and set aside.

1. Brown the chicken in the bacon fat. Remove from the pot.

1. Sauté the onion and garlic in the same pot.

1. Add the wine, broth, carrots, thyme, bay leaf, and chicken. Simmer for 1 hour.

1. Add the bacon back before serving.

Recipe 18: Ratatouille
Serves: 6 | **Prep Time:** 20 minutes | **Cook Time:** 45 minutes
Ingredients:

- 2 eggplants, diced

- 2 zucchini, sliced

- 1 onion, sliced

- 3 garlic cloves, minced

- 4 tomatoes, chopped

- 2 tbsp olive oil

- 1 tsp thyme

- Salt and pepper to taste

Instructions:

1. Heat olive oil in a pot. Sauté the onion and garlic for 5 minutes.

1. Add eggplant, zucchini, and tomatoes.

1. Season with thyme, salt, and pepper. Simmer for 45 minutes.

1. Serve warm with crusty bread.

Greek Cuisine

Recipe 19: Moussaka
Serves: 6 | **Prep Time:** 30 minutes | **Cook Time:** 1 hour
Ingredients:

- 2 eggplants, sliced

- 1 lb ground lamb

- 1 onion, chopped

- 1 tsp cinnamon

- 1 can (15 oz) tomatoes

- 1 cup béchamel sauce

- ½ cup Parmesan cheese

Instructions:

1. Sauté the lamb with onion and cinnamon. Add the tomatoes and simmer.

1. Layer eggplant slices and meat mixture in a baking dish.

1. Top with béchamel sauce and Parmesan. Bake at 375°F (190°C) for 1 hour.

Recipe 20: Spanakopita (Spinach Pie)
Serves: 8 | **Prep Time:** 30 minutes | **Cook Time:** 45 minutes
Ingredients:

- 1 lb spinach, chopped

- 1 onion, diced

- ½ cup feta cheese

- 8 sheets of phyllo dough

- ½ cup olive oil

Instructions:

1. Sauté the onion and spinach. Mix with feta cheese.

1. Layer phyllo dough, brush with olive oil between layers.

1. Add the spinach mixture and cover with more dough.

1. Bake at 375°F (190°C) for 45 minutes.

Thai Cuisine

Recipe 21: Green Curry with Vegetables

Serves: 4 | **Prep Time:** 15 minutes | **Cook Time:** 25 minutes

Ingredients:

- 2 tbsp green curry paste

- 1 can (15 oz) coconut milk

- 1 zucchini, sliced

- 1 bell pepper, sliced

- 1 cup broccoli florets

Instructions:

1. Heat the curry paste in a pan.

1. Add coconut milk and bring to a simmer.

1. Add the vegetables and cook for 10 minutes. Serve with jasmine rice.

Recipe 22: Pad Thai

Serves: 4 | **Prep Time:** 20 minutes | **Cook Time:** 10 minutes

Ingredients:

- 8 oz rice noodles

- 2 tbsp tamarind paste

- 2 tbsp fish sauce

- 1 tbsp sugar

- 2 eggs

- 1 cup bean sprouts

- Crushed peanuts

Instructions:

1. Cook the noodles according to package instructions.

1. Stir-fry the tamarind, fish sauce, and sugar. Add the eggs and scramble.

1. Toss in the noodles and sprouts. Top with peanuts.

Korean Cuisine

Recipe 23: Bulgogi (Korean BBQ Beef)
Serves: 4 | **Prep Time:** 15 minutes | **Cook Time:** 10 minutes
Ingredients:

- 1 lb thinly sliced beef

- ¼ cup soy sauce

- 2 tbsp sugar

- 2 garlic cloves, minced

- 1 tsp sesame oil

Instructions:

1. Marinate the beef in soy sauce, sugar, garlic, and sesame oil.

1. Grill or pan-fry for 5 minutes on each side.

Recipe 24: Bibimbap
Serves: 4 | **Prep Time:** 15 minutes | **Cook Time:** 10 minutes
Ingredients:

- 2 cups cooked rice

- 1 zucchini, sliced

- 1 carrot, julienned

- 4 fried eggs

- Gochujang sauce

Instructions:

1. Arrange the vegetables over the rice.

1. Top each bowl with a fried egg and drizzle with gochujang.

Japanese Cuisine

Recipe 25: Teriyaki Chicken

Serves: 4 | **Prep Time:** 10 minutes | **Cook Time:** 15 minutes

Ingredients:

- 4 chicken thighs

- ¼ cup soy sauce

- 2 tbsp honey

Instructions:

1. Marinate the chicken in soy sauce and honey.

1. Grill for 10 minutes.

Recipe 26: Miso Ramen

Serves: 4 | **Prep Time:** 10 minutes | **Cook Time:** 15 minutes

Ingredients:

- 4 cups of broth

- 2 tbsp miso paste

- 4 eggs, soft-boiled

Instructions:

1. Simmer the broth and miso.

1. Add the noodles and eggs.

Filipino Cuisine

Recipe 27: Chicken Adobo
Serves: 4 | **Prep Time:** 10 minutes | **Cook Time:** 30 minutes
Ingredients:

- 4 chicken thighs

- ¼ cup soy sauce

- ¼ cup vinegar

Instructions:

1. Simmer the chicken with soy sauce and vinegar for 30 minutes.

Recipe 28: Lumpia (Filipino Spring Rolls)
Serves: 6 | **Prep Time:** 30 minutes | **Cook Time:** 15 minutes
Ingredients:

- 1 lb ground pork

- 1 carrot, grated

- Lumpia wrappers

Instructions:

1. Roll the filling in wrappers. Fry until golden.

Turkish Cuisine

Recipe 29: Imam Bayildi (Stuffed Eggplant)
Serves: 4 | **Prep Time:** 20 minutes | **Cook Time:** 30 minutes
Instructions:

1. Stuff eggplants with tomatoes and onions.

1. Bake for 30 minutes.

Recipe 30: Kebab
Serves: 4 | **Cook Time:** 15 minutes
Instructions:

1. Grill seasoned lamb on skewers and enjoy!

Caribbean Cuisine

Recipe 31: Jamaican Brown Stew Chicken
Serves: 4 | **Prep Time:** 20 minutes | **Cook Time:** 1 hour
Ingredients:

- 2 lbs chicken thighs and drumsticks

- 2 tbsp of brown sugar

- 2 tbsp soy sauce

- 1 onion, sliced

- 2 garlic cloves, minced

- 1 bell pepper, sliced

- 1 cup chicken broth

- 1 tsp thyme

- 1 Scotch bonnet pepper (optional)

- Salt and pepper to taste

Instructions:

1. Rub the chicken with brown sugar and soy sauce. Let marinate for 30 minutes.

1. In a pan, brown the chicken on both sides. Set aside.

1. Sauté the onion, garlic, and bell pepper in the same pan.

1. Add the chicken back to the pan with broth, thyme, and Scotch

bonnet pepper.

1. Simmer for 40-45 minutes until the chicken is tender.

Recipe 32: Trinidadian Callaloo (Vegetable Stew)
Serves: 4 | **Prep Time:** 15 minutes | **Cook Time:** 30 minutes
Ingredients:

- 1 tbsp coconut oil

- 1 onion, diced

- 2 garlic cloves, minced

- 1 bunch spinach, chopped

- 1 can (15 oz) coconut milk

- 1 tsp thyme

- ½ tsp nutmeg

- Salt and pepper to taste

Instructions:

1. Heat the coconut oil and sauté the onion and garlic for 5 minutes.

1. Add the spinach and cook until wilted.

1. Pour in the coconut milk and season with thyme, nutmeg, salt, and pepper.

1. Simmer for 20 minutes and serve with rice or bread.

Ethiopian Cuisine

Recipe 33: Doro Wat (Spicy Chicken Stew)
Serves: 4 | **Prep Time:** 20 minutes | **Cook Time:** 1 hour
Ingredients:

- 4 chicken thighs

- 2 onions, finely chopped

- 2 tbsp ghee or clarified butter

- 2 garlic cloves, minced

- 1 tbsp berbere spice blend

- 1 cup chicken broth

- 2 boiled eggs

- Salt to taste

Instructions:

1. Sauté the onions in ghee until golden brown.

1. Add garlic and berbere spice and cook for 2 minutes.

1. Add the chicken and broth. Simmer for 45 minutes until tender.

1. Add the boiled eggs during the last 10 minutes. Serve with injera bread.

Recipe 34: Misir Wat (Spicy Red Lentil Stew)
Serves: 4 | **Prep Time:** 10 minutes | **Cook Time:** 40 minutes

Ingredients:

- 1 cup red lentils

- 1 onion, diced

- 2 garlic cloves, minced

- 2 tbsp ghee or clarified butter

- 1 tbsp berbere spice

- 4 cups vegetable broth

- Salt to taste

Instructions:

1. Sauté the onion and garlic in ghee for 5 minutes.

1. Add the berbere spice and cook for 1 minute.

1. Stir in the lentils and broth. Simmer for 30-35 minutes until the lentils are soft.

1. Serve with injera or rice.

Conclusion: A True Global Feast

With these final additions to your cuisines, your collection of entrées offers a taste of the world, reflecting the diversity and richness of global culinary traditions. These dishes not only celebrate tradition but also align with your goals for healthy, vibrant eating.

Up next: **Desserts**—sweet treats that indulge the senses without compromising health!

These culturally diverse entrées allow you to explore flavors from around the world while staying healthy and satisfied. Up next: **Desserts**—sweet treats that won't derail your health goals!

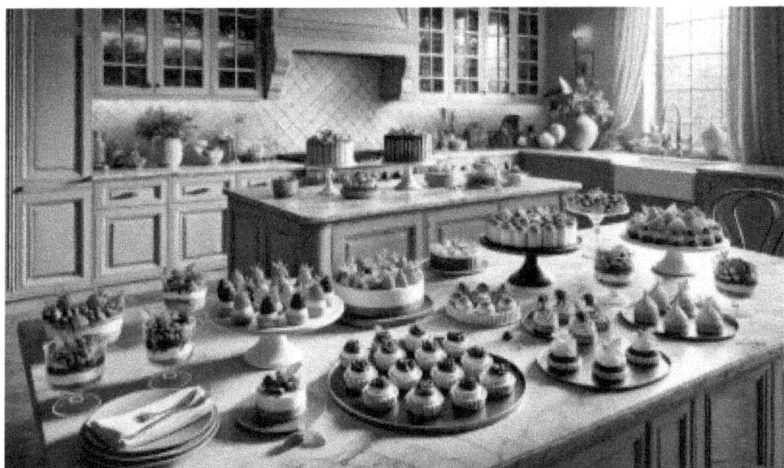

Part 2 Chapter 4: Decadent Desserts from Around the World

African Cuisine

Recipe 1: Malva Pudding (South African Caramel Cake)
Serves: 8 | **Prep Time:** 15 minutes | **Cook Time:** 45 minutes
Ingredients:

- 1 cup flour

- 1 tsp baking soda

- ½ cup sugar

- 1 egg

- 2 tbsp apricot jam

- 1 tbsp butter

- 1 cup milk

For the Sauce:

- ½ cup cream

- ½ cup sugar

- 2 tbsp butter

- 1 tsp vanilla

Instructions:

1. Preheat the oven to 350°F (175°C). Grease a baking dish.

1. In a bowl, mix the flour and baking soda. In another bowl, beat the egg, sugar, and apricot jam until light.

1. Melt the butter and add it to the egg mixture along with the milk. Mix well.

1. Gradually stir in the flour mixture. Pour into the baking dish and bake for 45 minutes.

1. For the sauce, heat the cream, sugar, butter, and vanilla in a saucepan until melted. Pour over the hot pudding.

Recipe 2: Moroccan Almond Cookies (Ghriba)
Serves: 12 | **Prep Time:** 15 minutes | **Cook Time:** 20 minutes
Ingredients:

- 2 cups almond flour

- 1 cup powdered sugar

- 2 eggs

- 1 tsp orange blossom water

Instructions:

1. Preheat the oven to 350°F (175°C). Line a baking sheet with parchment paper.

1. Mix the almond flour and powdered sugar in a bowl. Add the eggs and orange blossom water.

1. Shape the dough into small balls and flatten slightly.

1. Bake for 15-20 minutes until golden.

Italian Cuisine

Recipe 3: Tiramisu

Serves: 8 | **Prep Time:** 30 minutes | **Chill Time:** 4 hours

Ingredients:

- 2 cups espresso, cooled

- 24 ladyfingers

- 3 egg yolks

- ½ cup sugar

- 8 oz mascarpone cheese

- 1 cup heavy cream

- Cocoa powder for dusting

Instructions:

1. Whisk the egg yolks and sugar until pale. Add the mascarpone and mix until smooth.

1. In a separate bowl, whip the heavy cream to stiff peaks and fold into the mascarpone mixture.

1. Dip the ladyfingers in espresso and layer them in a dish. Spread half the mascarpone mixture over the ladyfingers. Repeat with another layer.

1. Chill for at least 4 hours. Dust with cocoa powder before serving.

Recipe 4: Italian Panna Cotta

Serves: 6 | **Prep Time:** 10 minutes | **Chill Time:** 4 hours

Ingredients:

- 2 cups of cream

- ½ cup sugar

- 1 tsp vanilla extract

- 1 packet of gelatin

Instructions:

1. Heat the cream, sugar, and vanilla in a saucepan until warm.

1. Dissolve the gelatin in 2 tbsp of water. Add to the cream mixture and stir until combined.

1. Pour into molds and chill for 4 hours. Serve with fresh fruit.

Mexican Cuisine

Recipe 5: Churros with Chocolate Sauce

Serves: 6 | **Prep Time:** 20 minutes | **Cook Time:** 15 minutes

Ingredients:

- 1 cup of water

- 2 tbsp sugar

- ½ tsp salt

- 1 cup flour

- 2 eggs

- Oil for frying

For the Chocolate Sauce:

- 1 cup dark chocolate

- ½ cup cream

Instructions:

1. Heat the water, sugar, and salt in a saucepan. Add the flour and stir until smooth.

1. Remove from heat and mix in the eggs. Transfer to a piping bag.

1. Heat oil and pipe the dough into the oil. Fry until golden.

1. Melt the chocolate with cream for the sauce. Serve churros with chocolate sauce.

Recipe 6: Flan (Mexican Caramel Custard)
Serves: 8 | **Prep Time:** 10 minutes | **Cook Time:** 50 minutes
Ingredients:

- 1 cup sugar

- 1 can (14 oz) sweetened condensed milk

- 1 can (12 oz) evaporated milk

- 3 eggs

- 1 tsp vanilla

Instructions:

1. Preheat the oven to 350°F (175°C).

1. Caramelize the sugar in a saucepan. Pour into a baking dish.

1. Blend the condensed milk, evaporated milk, eggs, and vanilla. Pour over the caramel.

1. Bake in a water bath for 50 minutes. Cool and invert to serve.

Indian Cuisine

Recipe 7: Gulab Jamun (Fried Dough Balls in Syrup)
Serves: 12 | **Prep Time:** 20 minutes | **Cook Time:** 15 minutes
Ingredients:

- 1 cup milk powder

- ¼ cup flour

- ¼ tsp baking soda

- 2 tbsp ghee

- ½ cup milk

For the Syrup:

- 2 cups of sugar

- 1 cup of water

- 1 tsp cardamom

Instructions:

1. Mix the dough ingredients and form small balls.

1. Fry the balls in ghee until golden.

1. Simmer sugar, water, and cardamom for 10 minutes to make syrup.

1. Soak the fried dough in syrup.

Recipe 8: Kheer (Indian Rice Pudding)

Serves: 6 | **Prep Time:** 10 minutes | **Cook Time:** 45 minutes

Ingredients:

- ½ cup basmati rice

- 4 cups milk

- ½ cup sugar

- 1 tsp cardamom

- 2 tbsp chopped nuts

Instructions:

1. Simmer the rice in milk until soft, about 40 minutes.

1. Add sugar, cardamom, and nuts. Cook for 5 more minutes.

Caribbean Cuisine

Recipe 9: Jamaican Rum Cake
Serves: 8 | **Prep Time:** 30 minutes | **Cook Time:** 1 hour
Ingredients:

- 2 cups of flour

- 1 cup sugar

- ½ cup butter

- 4 eggs

- ½ cup rum

- 1 tsp vanilla

Instructions:

1. Cream the butter and sugar. Add eggs and mix.

1. Add flour, rum, and vanilla. Mix until smooth.

1. Bake at 350°F (175°C) for 1 hour.

Recipe 10: Coconut Drops
Serves: 12 | **Prep Time:** 10 minutes | **Cook Time:** 20 minutes
Ingredients:

- 2 cups of shredded coconut

- 1 cup sugar

- 1 tsp ginger

- ½ cup water

Instructions:

1. Simmer all ingredients until thickened.

1. Drop spoonfuls onto a baking sheet and cool.

Ethiopian Cuisine

Recipe 11: Dabo Kolo (Sweet Fried Dough Bites)
Serves: 8 | **Prep Time:** 10 minutes | **Cook Time:** 15 minutes
Ingredients:

- 2 cups of flour

- ½ cup sugar

- 1 tsp cinnamon

- Oil for frying

Instructions:

1. Mix flour, sugar, and cinnamon.

1. Roll into small balls and fry until golden.

Recipe 12: Honey Cake (Ethiopian Tej Cake)
Serves: 8 | **Prep Time:** 15 minutes | **Cook Time:** 45 minutes
Ingredients:

- 2 cups of flour

- ½ cup honey

- 1 tsp baking soda

- 1 tsp cinnamon

Instructions:

1. Mix the ingredients and pour into a greased pan.

1. Bake at 350°F (175°C) for 45 minutes.

Middle Eastern Cuisine

Recipe 1: Baklava

Serves: 12 | **Prep Time:** 30 minutes | **Cook Time:** 1 hour

Ingredients:

- 1 package phyllo dough

- 2 cups chopped walnuts

- 1 tsp cinnamon

- 1 cup butter, melted

- 1 cup sugar

- ½ cup honey

- ½ cup water

- 1 tsp lemon juice

Instructions:

1. Preheat the oven to 350°F (175°C).

1. Mix the walnuts and cinnamon.

1. Brush a baking dish with melted butter and layer 8 sheets of phyllo, brushing each with butter.

1. Add a layer of the walnut mixture and continue layering phyllo and walnuts.

1. Bake for 50 minutes until golden.

1. Boil sugar, honey, water, and lemon juice to make the syrup. Pour over the warm baklava.

Recipe 2: Basbousa (Semolina Cake)
Serves: 10 | **Prep Time:** 15 minutes | **Cook Time:** 30 minutes
Ingredients:

- 1½ cups semolina

- ½ cup sugar

- 1 tsp baking powder

- ½ cup plain yogurt

- ½ cup melted butter

- ½ cup almonds

For the Syrup:

- 1 cup sugar

- ½ cup water

- 1 tsp lemon juice

Instructions:

1. Preheat the oven to 350°F (175°C). Mix semolina, sugar, baking powder, yogurt, and butter.

1. Pour into a greased dish and top with almonds.

1. Bake for 30 minutes.

1. Boil the syrup ingredients and pour over the cake while warm.

Chinese Cuisine

Recipe 3: Mango Pudding
Serves: 6 | **Prep Time:** 15 minutes | **Chill Time:** 2 hours
Ingredients:

- 2 ripe mangoes, pureed

- 1 cup milk

- ½ cup sugar

- 1 packet gelatin

- ½ cup hot water

Instructions:

1. Dissolve the gelatin in hot water.

1. Mix the mango puree, milk, and sugar.

1. Stir in the gelatin and pour into molds.

1. Chill for at least 2 hours before serving.

Recipe 4: Sesame Balls (Jian Dui)
Serves: 8 | **Prep Time:** 30 minutes | **Cook Time:** 15 minutes
Ingredients:

- 2 cups glutinous rice flour

- ½ cup sugar

- ¾ cup water

- Red bean paste

- Sesame seeds

- Oil for frying

Instructions:

1. Mix the rice flour, sugar, and water to form a dough.

1. Divide into small balls and fill with red bean paste.

1. Roll in sesame seeds and fry until golden.

Korean Cuisine

Recipe 5: Hotteok (Sweet Pancakes)
Serves: 8 | **Prep Time:** 1 hour | **Cook Time:** 10 minutes
Ingredients:

- 2 cups of flour

- 2 tbsp sugar

- 1 tsp yeast

- ¾ cup warm milk

- ½ cup brown sugar

- 1 tsp cinnamon

Instructions:

1. Mix flour, sugar, yeast, and milk to form a dough. Let rise for 1 hour.

1. Roll into balls and fill with brown sugar and cinnamon.

1. Flatten and pan-fry until golden.

Recipe 6: Yakgwa (Honey Cookies)
Serves: 12 | **Prep Time:** 30 minutes | **Cook Time:** 15 minutes
Ingredients:

- 2 cups flour

- ½ cup sesame oil

- ½ cup honey

- ½ cup water

Instructions:

1. Mix flour and sesame oil. Add honey and water to form dough.

1. Roll out and cut into shapes.

1. Fry until golden.

Japanese Cuisine

Recipe 7: Mochi (Glutinous Rice Cakes)
Serves: 12 | **Prep Time:** 20 minutes | **Cook Time:** 10 minutes
Ingredients:

- 1 cup glutinous rice flour

- ½ cup sugar

- 1 cup water

- Red bean paste

Instructions:

1. Mix the flour, sugar, and water.

1. Microwave for 2 minutes, stir, and microwave for 1 more minute.

1. Divide the dough and fill with red bean paste.

Recipe 8: Matcha Ice Cream
Serves: 4 | **Prep Time:** 10 minutes | **Churn Time:** 30 minutes
Ingredients:

- 2 cups heavy cream

- 1 cup milk

- ½ cup sugar

- 2 tbsp matcha powder

Instructions:

1. Whisk the sugar and matcha with milk and cream.

1. Pour into an ice cream maker and churn for 30 minutes.

French Cuisine

Recipe 9: Crème Brûlée
Serves: 6 | **Prep Time:** 15 minutes | **Cook Time:** 30 minutes
Ingredients:

- 2 cups heavy cream

- ½ cup sugar

- 4 egg yolks

- 1 tsp vanilla extract

- Sugar for caramelizing

Instructions:

1. Preheat the oven to 325°F (160°C).

1. Heat the cream. Whisk the yolks, sugar, and vanilla.

1. Slowly add the cream to the yolks. Pour into ramekins.

1. Bake for 30 minutes. Chill, then caramelize the tops with sugar.

Recipe 10: Profiteroles
Serves: 8 | **Prep Time:** 20 minutes | **Cook Time:** 30 minutes
Ingredients:

- 1 cup water

- ½ cup butter

- 1 cup flour

- 4 eggs

- Whipped cream for filling

- Chocolate sauce

Instructions:

1. Boil water and butter. Add flour and stir.

1. Add eggs one at a time. Pipe onto a baking sheet.

1. Bake at 400°F (200°C) for 20 minutes. Fill with cream and top with chocolate sauce.

Greek Cuisine

Recipe 11: Loukoumades (Honey Doughnuts)
Serves: 8 | **Prep Time:** 30 minutes | **Cook Time:** 15 minutes
Ingredients:

- 2 cups flour

- 1 tsp yeast

- ¾ cup warm water

- Honey for drizzling

Instructions:

1. Mix flour, yeast, and water. Let rise for 1 hour.

1. Fry spoonfuls of dough until golden. Drizzle with honey.

Recipe 12: Greek Yogurt with Honey and Nuts
Serves: 4 | **Prep Time:** 5 minutes
Ingredients:

- 2 cups Greek yogurt

- ¼ cup honey

- ½ cup walnuts

Instructions:

1. Divide yogurt into bowls.

1. Drizzle with honey and top with walnuts.

146

Thai Cuisine

Recipe 13: Sticky Rice with Mango
Serves: 4 | **Prep Time:** 15 minutes | **Cook Time:** 30 minutes
Ingredients:

- 1 cup sticky rice

- 1 cup coconut milk

- ¼ cup sugar

- 2 ripe mangoes

Instructions:

1. Cook the sticky rice. Mix coconut milk and sugar and stir into the rice.

1. Serve with sliced mango.

Recipe 14: Thai Coconut Custard
Serves: 6 | **Prep Time:** 10 minutes | **Cook Time:** 20 minutes
Ingredients:

- 1 cup coconut milk

- ½ cup sugar

- 4 eggs

Instructions:

1. Mix all ingredients. Pour into molds.

1. Steam for 20 minutes.

Filipino Cuisine

Recipe 15: Halo-Halo
Serves: 4 | **Prep Time:** 15 minutes
Ingredients:

- Shaved ice

- Sweet beans

- Ice cream

- Fruit toppings

Instructions:

1. Layer all ingredients in a tall glass.

Recipe 16: Leche Flan
Serves: 8 | **Prep Time:** 10 minutes | **Cook Time:** 50 minutes
Instructions:

1. Caramelize sugar. Pour into a dish.

1. Blend condensed milk, eggs, and evaporated milk.

1. Bake for 50 minutes in a water bath.

Turkish Cuisine

Recipe 17: Turkish Delight
    Serves: 12 | **Prep Time:** 30 minutes
    Instructions:

1. Simmer sugar and cornstarch to form candy.

Recipe 18: Kunafa
    Instructions:

1. Layer shredded pastry with cheese. Bake and drizzle with syrup.

Conclusion: A Sweet Ending to Complete Your Global Feast

These desserts take you on a flavorful journey through the sweet traditions of the world. From light puddings to rich cakes, there's something for everyone to indulge in without guilt. With the addition of these diverse desserts, every culture from the entrée section is now paired with a complementary sweet treat. This ensures you can create cohesive, culturally authentic meals—from savory to sweet—offering a complete culinary experience.

Up next: Snacks from Around the World—quick, healthy bites to fuel your day and keep you energized between meals.

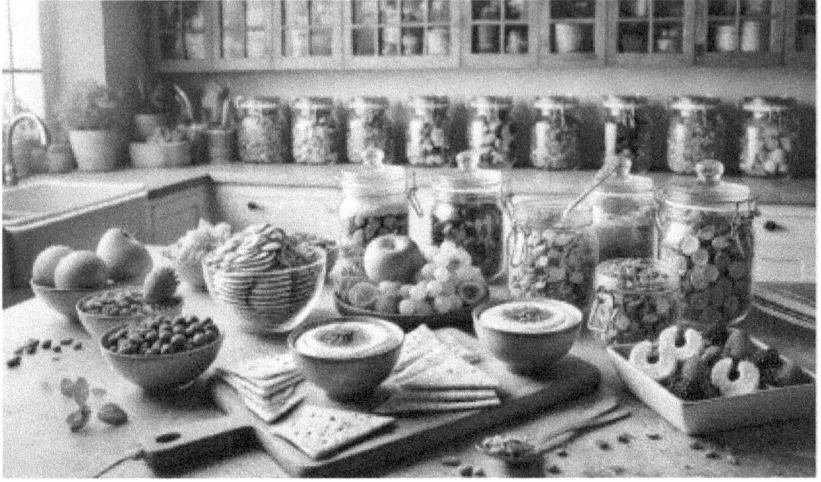

Part 2 Chapter 5: Healthy Snacks from Around the World

African Cuisine

Recipe 1: Spicy Plantain Chips
Serves: 4 | **Prep Time:** 10 minutes | **Cook Time:** 15 minutes
Ingredients:

- 2 green plantains

- 1 tsp cayenne pepper

- 1 tsp of salt

- 2 tbsp olive oil

Instructions:

1. Preheat the oven to 375°F (190°C).

1. Peel and slice the plantains into thin rounds.

1. Toss with olive oil, cayenne, and salt.

1. Spread on a baking sheet and bake for 15 minutes until crispy.

Recipe 2: Roasted Chickpeas
Serves: 4 | **Prep Time:** 10 minutes | **Cook Time:** 25 minutes
Ingredients:

- 1 can (15 oz) chickpeas, drained

- 2 tbsp olive oil

- 1 tsp paprika

- ½ tsp cumin

Instructions:

1. Preheat the oven to 400°F (200°C).

1. Toss the chickpeas with olive oil and spices.

1. Roast for 20-25 minutes until crispy.

Italian Cuisine

Recipe 3: Caprese Skewers
Serves: 8 | **Prep Time:** 10 minutes
Ingredients:

- Cherry tomatoes

- Fresh mozzarella balls

- Fresh basil leaves

- Balsamic glaze

Instructions:

1. Thread a tomato, mozzarella ball, and basil leaf onto each skewer.

1. Drizzle with balsamic glaze before serving.

Recipe 4: Bruschetta with Tomato and Basil
Serves: 6 | **Prep Time:** 10 minutes | **Cook Time:** 5 minutes
Ingredients:

- 1 baguette, sliced

- 2 tomatoes, diced

- 2 tbsp olive oil

- 1 garlic clove, minced

- Fresh basil, chopped

Instructions:

1. Toast the baguette slices until golden.

1. Mix the tomatoes, garlic, olive oil, and basil.

1. Spoon the mixture onto the toasted bread.

Mexican Cuisine

Recipe 5: Guacamole with Veggie Sticks
Serves: 4 | **Prep Time:** 10 minutes
Ingredients:

- 2 ripe avocados

- 1 lime, juiced

- 1 small onion, diced

- Salt to taste

- Carrot and celery sticks

Instructions:

1. Mash the avocados with lime juice, onion, and salt.

1. Serve with veggie sticks for dipping.

Recipe 6: Spiced Pumpkin Seeds (Pepitas)
Serves: 4 | **Prep Time:** 5 minutes | **Cook Time:** 15 minutes
Ingredients:

- 1 cup of pumpkin seeds

- 1 tbsp olive oil

- 1 tsp chili powder

- Salt to taste

Instructions:

1. Preheat the oven to 350°F (175°C).

1. Toss the pumpkin seeds with oil, chili powder, and salt.

1. Roast for 10-15 minutes until crispy.

Indian Cuisine

Recipe 7: Masala Popcorn
Serves: 4 | **Prep Time:** 5 minutes | **Cook Time:** 5 minutes
Ingredients:

- ½ cup popcorn kernels

- 2 tbsp coconut oil

- 1 tsp garam masala

Instructions:

1. Pop the kernels in coconut oil.

1. Sprinkle with garam masala and toss well.

Recipe 8: Roasted Spiced Nuts
Serves: 4 | **Prep Time:** 5 minutes | **Cook Time:** 10 minutes
Ingredients:

- 2 cups of mixed nuts

- 1 tbsp ghee

- 1 tsp cumin

- ½ tsp turmeric

Instructions:

1. Heat ghee in a pan and toast the nuts with spices for 10 minutes.

Greek Cuisine

Recipe 9: Greek Yogurt Parfaits
Serves: 4 | **Prep Time:** 10 minutes
Ingredients:

- 2 cups Greek yogurt

- 1 cup granola

- ½ cup mixed berries

Instructions:

1. Layer yogurt, granola, and berries in small glasses or bowls.

Recipe 10: Cucumber Hummus Bites
Serves: 6 | **Prep Time:** 10 minutes
Ingredients:

- 2 cucumbers, sliced

- ½ cup hummus

- Paprika for garnish

Instructions:

1. Spread hummus on each cucumber slice.

1. Sprinkle with paprika and serve.

Thai Cuisine

Recipe 11: Fresh Spring Rolls
Serves: 6 | **Prep Time:** 20 minutes
Ingredients:

- Rice paper wrappers

- Lettuce leaves

- Shredded carrots

- Mint leaves

- Sweet chili sauce

Instructions:

1. Soak the rice paper wrappers in water until soft.

1. Fill with lettuce, carrots, and mint. Roll tightly and serve with chili sauce.

Recipe 12: Mango Slices with Lime and Chili
Serves: 4 | **Prep Time:** 5 minutes
Ingredients:

- 2 ripe mangoes, sliced

- 1 lime, juiced

- Chili powder to taste

Instructions:

1. Drizzle lime juice over the mango slices.

1. Sprinkle with chili powder before serving.

Japanese Cuisine

Recipe 13: Edamame with Sea Salt
Serves: 4 | **Prep Time:** 5 minutes | **Cook Time:** 5 minutes
Ingredients:

- 2 cups of edamame

- Sea salt to taste

Instructions:

1. Boil the edamame for 5 minutes.

1. Sprinkle with sea salt and serve.

Recipe 14: Rice Crackers (Senbei)
Serves: 6 | **Prep Time:** 15 minutes | **Cook Time:** 10 minutes
Ingredients:

- 2 cups of cooked rice

- 1 tbsp soy sauce

Instructions:

1. Shape the rice into small patties.

1. Brush with soy sauce and bake at 350°F (175°C) for 10 minutes.

Turkish Cuisine

Recipe 15: Roasted Chestnuts
Serves: 6 | **Prep Time:** 10 minutes | **Cook Time:** 25 minutes
Ingredients:

- 2 lbs chestnuts

Instructions:

1. Cut an X into each chestnut.

1. Roast at 400°F (200°C) for 25 minutes.

Recipe 16: Yogurt and Cucumber Dip (Cacik)
Serves: 4 | **Prep Time:** 10 minutes
Ingredients:

- 1 cup yogurt

- 1 cucumber, grated

- 1 garlic clove, minced

- Mint for garnish

Instructions:

1. Mix the yogurt, cucumber, and garlic.

1. Garnish with mint and serve.

Conclusion: Snack Smart, Snack Global

With these healthy snacks from around the world, you have plenty of options to keep you energized throughout the day. Each snack offers unique flavors, reflecting the culinary heritage of its culture while supporting your health goals.

Up next: **Smoothies**—power-packed drinks to start your day right or refuel after a workout!

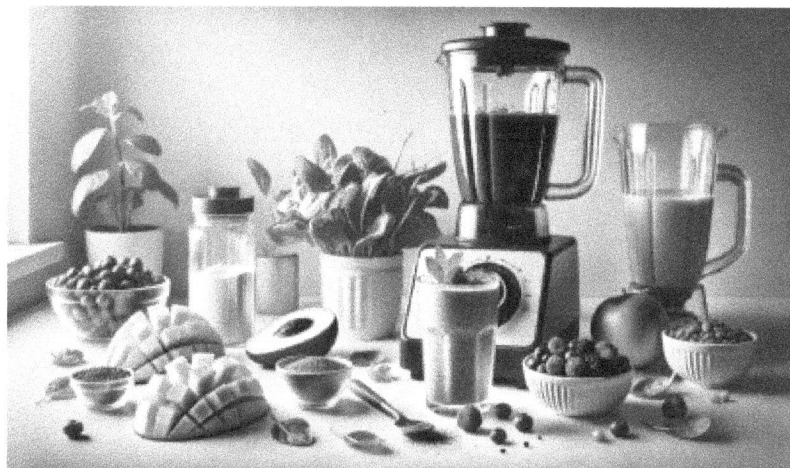

Chapter 6: Smoothies from Around the World

African-Inspired Smoothies

Recipe 1: Tropical Mango and Pineapple Smoothie
Serves: 2 | **Prep Time:** 5 minutes
Ingredients:

- 1 cup mango chunks (fresh or frozen)

- 1 cup of pineapple chunks

- 1 banana

- ½ cup coconut water

- 1 tbsp chia seeds

Instructions:

1. Add all the ingredients to the blender.

1. Blend until smooth and creamy.

1. Serve chilled.

Recipe 2: Hibiscus and Watermelon Smoothie
Serves: 2 | **Prep Time:** 10 minutes
Ingredients:

- 2 cups of watermelon, cubed

- ½ cup hibiscus tea, cooled

- 1 tbsp lime juice

- 1 tsp honey (optional)

Instructions:

1. Combine all the ingredients in a blender.

1. Blend until smooth.

1. Serve over ice.

Italian-Inspired Smoothies

Recipe 3: Berry and Yogurt Smoothie
Serves: 2 | **Prep Time:** 5 minutes
Ingredients:

- 1 cup mixed berries (strawberries, blueberries, raspberries)

- ½ cup plain Greek yogurt

- ½ cup almond milk

- 1 tsp honey

Instructions:

1. Blend all ingredients until smooth.

1. Garnish with fresh berries.

Recipe 4: Espresso and Banana Smoothie
Serves: 2 | **Prep Time:** 5 minutes
Ingredients:

- 1 banana

- ½ cup brewed espresso, chilled

- ½ cup oat milk

- 1 tsp cocoa powder

Instructions:

1. Blend until smooth.

1. Serve with a dusting of cocoa powder.

Mexican-Inspired Smoothies

Recipe 5: Avocado and Lime Smoothie
Serves: 2 | **Prep Time:** 5 minutes
Ingredients:

- 1 avocado

- 1 cup almond milk

- 2 tbsp lime juice

- 1 tsp honey

Instructions:

1. Blend all ingredients until creamy.

1. Serve chilled.

Recipe 6: Horchata Smoothie
Serves: 2 | **Prep Time:** 5 minutes
Ingredients:

- 1 cup rice milk

- 1 tsp cinnamon

- 2 dates, pitted

- 1 frozen banana

Instructions:

1. Blend all ingredients until smooth.

1. Sprinkle with cinnamon before serving.

Indian-Inspired Smoothies

Recipe 7: Mango Lassi
   Serves: 2 | **Prep Time:** 5 minutes
   Ingredients:

- 1 cup mango chunks

- ½ cup plain yogurt

- ½ cup milk

- 1 tsp cardamom

Instructions:

1. Blend all ingredients until smooth.

1. Serve chilled.

Recipe 8: Turmeric Ginger Smoothie
Serves: 2 | **Prep Time:** 5 minutes
Ingredients:

- 1 banana

- 1 tsp turmeric

- ½ tsp grated ginger

- 1 cup coconut milk

Instructions:

1. Blend until creamy.

1. Serve with a sprinkle of turmeric.

Greek-Inspired Smoothies

Recipe 9: Cucumber and Mint Smoothie
Serves: 2 | **Prep Time:** 5 minutes
Ingredients:

- 1 cucumber, sliced

- ½ cup Greek yogurt

- 1 tbsp mint leaves

- ½ cup water

Instructions:

1. Blend until smooth.

1. Serve with a mint garnish.

Recipe 10: Honey and Walnut Smoothie
Serves: 2 | **Prep Time:** 5 minutes
Ingredients:

- 1 banana

- ½ cup Greek yogurt

- 1 tbsp honey

- 2 tbsp walnuts

Instructions:

1. Blend until creamy.

1. Garnish with crushed walnuts.

Japanese-Inspired Smoothies

Recipe 11: Matcha Green Smoothie
    Serves: 2 | **Prep Time:** 5 minutes
    Ingredients:

- 1 tsp matcha powder

- 1 banana

- 1 cup almond milk

- 1 tsp honey

Instructions:

1. Blend until smooth.

1. Serve with a sprinkle of matcha.

Recipe 12: Strawberry Tofu Smoothie
    Serves: 2 | **Prep Time:** 5 minutes
    Ingredients:

- 1 cup of strawberries

- ½ cup silken tofu

- 1 tsp vanilla extract

- 1 cup soy milk

Instructions:

1. Blend until smooth.

1. Garnish with sliced strawberries.

Thai-Inspired Smoothies

Recipe 13: Coconut Pineapple Smoothie
　　Serves: 2 | **Prep Time:** 5 minutes
　　Ingredients:

- 1 cup of pineapple chunks

- ½ cup coconut milk

- 1 tbsp shredded coconut

- Ice cubes

Instructions:

1. Blend until smooth.

1. Serve with shredded coconut.

Recipe 14: Thai Iced Tea Smoothie
　　Serves: 2 | **Prep Time:** 10 minutes
　　Ingredients:

- 1 cup brewed Thai tea, chilled

- ½ cup coconut milk

- 1 tbsp condensed milk

- Ice cubes

Instructions:

1. Blend until smooth.

1. Serve with a drizzle of condensed milk.

Conclusion: Smoothies for Every Occasion

These smoothies not only reflect the unique flavors of the cultures they come from but also offer a nutritious way to stay energized throughout the day. From tropical delights to creamy classics, each smoothie brings something special to your **NEW HEALTHY KITCHEN**.

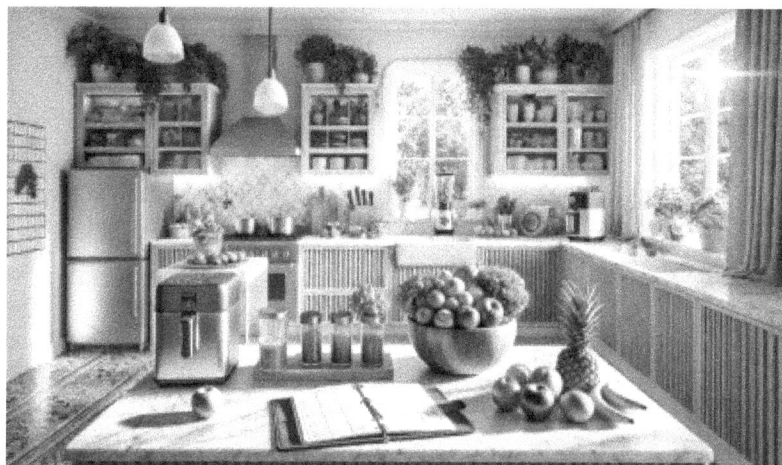

Part Three: Conclusion and Reflections – The Beginning of a Lifelong Journey

Introduction: Your Journey Doesn't End Here

Congratulations! You've taken a deep dive into building a healthy kitchen and explored how food connects us to cultures, traditions, and well-being. With knowledge, tools, recipes, and new habits at your disposal, you're now equipped to nourish yourself and those you care about. However, this is just the beginning. True wellness is a lifelong journey of learning, adapting, and celebrating the process.

Your kitchen has become more than a place to prepare meals—it's now a space for creativity, connection, and intentional living. As you've learned, eating well doesn't mean giving up flavor or joy; it means discovering new ways to enjoy food that fuels both your body and soul.

Sustaining the Change: Practical Tips for Moving Forward

1. Plan and Evolve
   Meal planning doesn't have to be rigid. Continue to explore new flavors, seasonal produce, and global recipes. Let your kitchen evolve with your preferences and health needs over time.

1. Practice Grace with Yourself
   Not every day will be perfect, and that's okay. Allow room for indulgence, learning, and mistakes. What matters most is consistency and intention, not perfection.

1. Involve Loved Ones
   A healthy kitchen can bring people together. Involve family and friends in cooking, sharing meals, and trying new recipes. These shared experiences build community and make the journey enjoyable.

1. Keep Learning
   The world of food is endless. Continue learning about nutrition, wellness, and different cuisines. Whether through cooking classes, books, or conversations with others, keep exploring.

Reflection: Food as More Than Fuel

Throughout this journey, you've discovered that food is much more than just fuel—it's culture, memory, tradition, and a way to connect with others. From the warmth of a comforting soup to the excitement of discovering a new snack, your meals tell stories. They reflect who you are and who you aspire to be.

As you've seen from the diverse range of recipes, there's beauty in variety. Each meal is an opportunity to celebrate life, honor heritage, and nourish your body. Whether you're creating something simple or preparing an elaborate feast, every dish carries meaning.

A Call to Action: Sharing Your Journey

Now that your kitchen is a place of health, joy, and creativity, consider how you can share your journey with others. Host a dinner party, teach a friend to make one of your favorite dishes, or donate meals to those in need. Food has the power to heal and connect, and by sharing what you've learned, you can inspire others to embark on their own healthy kitchen journey.

Final Encouragement: Keep Moving Forward

Building a healthy kitchen is not the end—it's the foundation for a healthier, happier life. Continue experimenting, savoring, and growing. Use the recipes and tools in this book as a starting point, but don't be afraid to chart your own path. Embrace every step of the way, knowing that each meal you create brings you closer to a life of wellness.

Remember, progress is not measured by perfection but by the small, daily choices that align with your goals. Whether it's enjoying a vibrant salad, savoring a decadent dessert, or sharing a simple meal with loved ones, every step forward matters.

Thank you for allowing this book to be part of your journey. May your kitchen always be filled with the warmth of good food, the joy of shared meals, and the love that comes from nourishing yourself and others.

Conclusion: A New Chapter Begins

As you close this book, know that you've created a powerful foundation for change. What lies ahead is a journey filled with discovery, joy, and health. Your kitchen is now a place where good habits thrive, cultural traditions are celebrated, and healthy living is embraced.

Here's to your fresh start, new beginnings, and the exciting journey ahead. May every forkful be a step toward the life you envision.

Thank You for Choosing a Healthier Life

Thank you for purchasing *Fridge, Forks, and Fresh Starts: Building a Healthy Kitchen* and for taking this important step toward a healthier, more vibrant lifestyle. I am honored that you've allowed this book to be part of your journey. It's not just about what you eat, but how you prepare, plan, and align your choices to create sustainable health for yourself and those around you.

Together, we are building the tools for success—starting in the kitchen—and I am grateful to walk alongside you. May the insights and strategies in these pages inspire and empower you to embrace lasting wellness and enjoy the process along the way.

Blessings on your journey,

Apostle Paula Ferguson

Don't miss out!

Visit the website below and you can sign up to receive emails whenever Apostle Paula Ferguson publishes a new book. There's no charge and no obligation.

https://books2read.com/r/B-A-EDXVD-DHFHH

BOOKS 2 READ

Connecting independent readers to independent writers.

Did you love *Fridge, Forks, and Fresh Starts: Building a Healthy Kitchen*? Then you should read *Arsenal: Prayers Declarations and Decrees That Will Move Heaven and Shake Hell*[1] by Apostle Paula Ferguson!

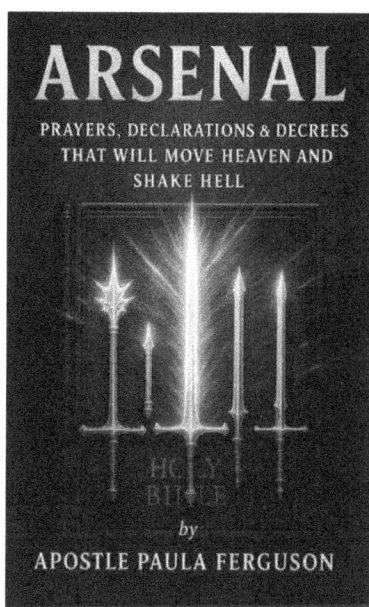

In an age where darkness assaults every stronghold—families torn by division, finances gripped by scarcity, and souls entangled by unseen forces—*Arsenal: Prayers, Declarations, and Decrees That Will Move Heaven and Shake Hell* by Apostle Paula Ferguson emerges as a divine imperative, a sacred armory that is not an option but a **REQUIREMENT** for every believer. This is no ordinary book; it is a celestial war chest, an apostolic mandate wielding 323 Spirit-breathed proclamations to dismantle strongholds, restore legacies, and align earth with Heaven's glory. Your victory will not come by wishful thinking; it will only come by decree! Open your mouth and SPEAK!

Forged under Apostle Ferguson's apostolic anointing, shaped by her mentors—Apostle Craig Ferguson, her steadfast husband; Denise Michelle Ray, her intercessor; Apostle Douglas Dwayne Rudd Sr., her spiritual father;

---

1. https://books2read.com/u/bQz9gd

2. https://books2read.com/u/bQz9gd

Prophet Lovy L. Elias, her prayer mentor; and Prophetess Taryn Nicole Bishop, her spiritual mother—*Arsenal* equips you with precision across 18 battlegrounds, from *Family Restoration* to the groundbreaking *Technological Warfare and Protection*. Rooted in over 150 Scriptures, each decree is a divine edict. Proclaim, "I decree that my marriage is fortified by divine love" (Chapter 1, #7), and watch unity prevail. Declare, "I decree that no algorithm invades my destiny" (Chapter 11, #16), and see God's shield rise. Whether a new believer sowing faith or a prayer general commanding Heaven's armies, this book is your non-negotiable weapon to co-create with God.

Apostle Ferguson's testimony—miracles of healed bodies, shifted policies, transformed lives—infuses *Arsenal* with unyielding power. Uniting African, Hispanic, Asian, and global believers, it transcends cultures in a universal call to arms. Morning Warfare Prayer Points and a Scripture Index ensure daily conquest, while vivid metaphors—your voice as a divine scepter, decrees as heavenly prescriptions—make truth accessible. This book is a **REQUIREMENT** to stand as a joint-heir with Christ (Romans 8:17), wielding your tongue's power (Proverbs 18:21) to break chains and spark revival. You cannot face this hour unarmed. Embrace *Arsenal*. Move Heaven. Shake Hell.

Read more at www.fosaservices.com.

Also by Apostle Paula Ferguson

Arsenal: Prayers Declarations and Decrees That Will Move Heaven and Shake Hell

Bag Lady, Mr. Bojangles: It's Time to Let It Go

Fridge, Forks, and Fresh Starts: Building a Healthy Kitchen

Watch for more at www.fosaservices.com.

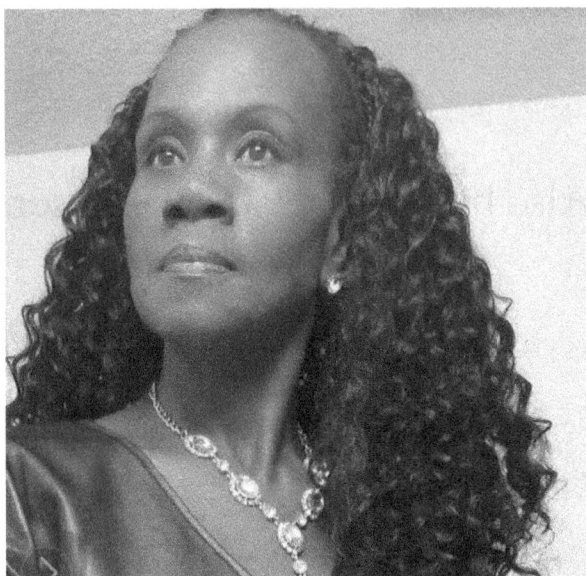

About the Author

Apostle Paula Ferguson is a dynamic prophetic leader, teacher, and author with decades of ministry experience, dedicated to empowering believers to walk boldly in their God-given authority. Known for her profound spiritual insight and unwavering commitment to biblical truth, she equips the body of Christ to break strongholds, shift atmospheres, and manifest God's promises through faith-filled declarations. Her ministry is marked by testimonies of healing, deliverance, and restoration, as she guides others to align their lives with Heaven's purposes.

As the author of *Bag Lady, Mr. Bojangles: It's Time to Let It Go*, *Make It Make Sense*, and *I Just Don't Feel Like It! Finding Motivation When Life Hits Snooze*, Apostle Paula combines real-life stories, scriptural wisdom, and practical steps to inspire transformation. She describes herself as a "human computer," receiving divine downloads from God to navigate life's challenges, a testimony woven throughout her writings and teachings.

Married to her best friend and greatest supporter, Apostle Craig Ferguson, she serves alongside him to foster spiritual growth, emotional healing, and holistic wellness. Together, they empower individuals to recognize their worth in Christ and embrace their divine purpose. Apostle Paula's transparent, compassionate approach and apostolic anointing make her a trusted voice for those seeking to move heaven and shake hell.

Read more at www.fosaservices.com.

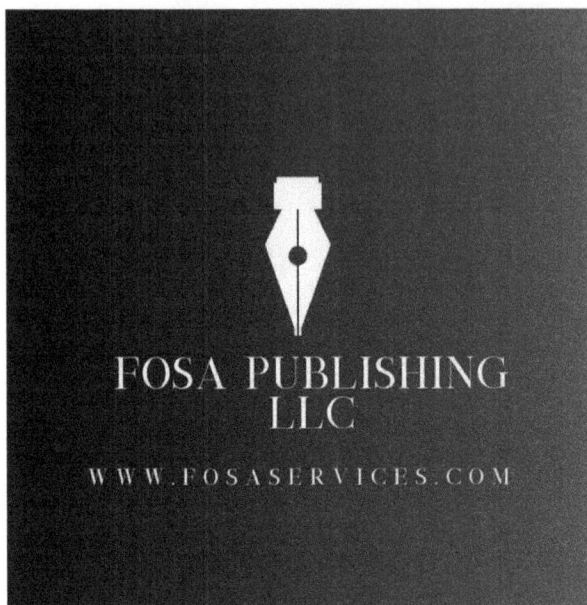

About the Publisher

FOSA Publishing LLC—short for *Family of Successful Authors*—is dedicated to empowering writers from all backgrounds to bring their stories to life. While our roots are in Christian publishing, we proudly support authors of diverse genres and messages.

Inspired by stories of perseverance, we aim to support authors in publishing their messages quickly and effectively. Our encouragement is simple: start where you are, trust your vision, and let us help you bring it to life.

Join our family of successful authors—your voice deserves to be heard.

Read more at https://fosaservices.com/.